A
VEGETARIAN
DOCTOR
SPEAKS
OUT

A VEGETARIAN DOCTOR SPEAKS OUT

Charles R. Attwood, M.D., F.A.A.P.

HOHM PRESS
PRESCOTT, AZ
1998

Cover design: Kim Johansen
Layout and design: Bhadra Mitchell,
Boulder, Colorado

Library of Congress Cataloging in Publication Data:

Attwood, Charles R.
   A vegetarian doctor speaks out / Charles R.
   Attwood
   p. cm.
   Includes bibliographical references and
   index
   ISBN 0-934252-85-8
   1. Vegetarianism. I. Title.
RM236.A88 1998
613.2'62--dc21   98-29999
                                                   CIP

Hohm Press
P.O. Box 2501
Prescott, AZ 86302
800-381-2700
http://www.booknotes.com/hohm/

To Judy,
my wife, companion and collaborator,
who has made this journey a festival.

CONTENTS

Acknowledgements

A very special thank-you to Jeff and Sabrina Nelson of VegSource . . . *http: www.vegsource.com/* . . . for their research assistance, support and friendship. Also to Tony Zuccarello and Regina Sara Ryan of Hohm Press for their enthusiasm for the information contained in these pages. And to my wife, Judy, for her thorough editing of the first draft. Finally, to my dear friends: T. Colin Campbell, Ph.D.; Caldwell Esselstyn, M.D. and the late Dr. Benjamin Spock. And finally, a special thanks to Pattie Breitman.

Preface

During the last two decades, a small group of professionals, an elite new breed, has emerged upon the national and international scene. These outspoken men and women, who have been referred to as "nutrition activists," have been extolling the health risks of eating a meat- and dairy-based diet, especially, focusing on the strong relationship between animal fat and protein to heart disease, stroke, diabetes and cancer.

This nutrition revolution gained even greater momentum during the 1990s, largely due to the relentless and enthusiastic writing and "speaking out" by these new leaders throughout the country. Not surprisingly, they have been called "nutrition terrorists" by the National Dairy Council and the National Beef Industry Council, both of which were concerned enough to launch new promotional efforts for their products—the best known is the celebrity "Milk Mustache" ads and billboards. Ironically, over forty years ago, the tobacco industry followed this general promotional scenario when the health risk of its products was becoming known.

I am honored to have worked along with this diverse and dedicated group of pioneers, who've shown such rare strength and vision at this time and place in our history. The giants among them are Neal Barnard, M.D, T. Colin Campbell, Ph.D., William Castelli, M.D., Caldwell Esselstyn, M.D., Suzanne Havala, M.S, R.D., Michael Klaper, M.D., John McDougall, M.D., Dean Ornish, M.D. and the late Benjamin Spock, M.D.

Where there is not vision, the people perish.
—Proverbs, 29:18

Introduction

A Torch of Knowledge

Something happened during the spring of 1995 that would change my life forever. My solo pediatric practice had become, according to the *Medical Economics Magazine,* one of the most lucrative in the nation, with gross earnings reaching $1,200,000 annually. As a solo doctor, board-certified in my specialty, I was seeing up to ninety patients each day with the help of a devoted, hardworking staff of ten. The practice was so successful, I had begun writing articles about it for medical practice management magazines, including a series of ten essays for *Medical Economics.* One of these, an article about Medicaid, won a national first place award for the magazine in 1991.

In March 1995, my book on nutrition, *Dr. Attwood's Low-Fat Prescription for Kids,* which I had spent five years researching and writing during evenings and weekends, was published by Viking-Penguin. I hired another doctor to take care of my practice while I went on the road for a national, two-week, book promotional tour arranged by my publisher. But I never returned.

Incredibly, that book tour was to become an ongoing international lecture tour, during which I would be speaking in over two hundred cities (and counting) at universities, corporate conferences, environmental organizations, medical and health organizations, education groups, professional conferences, churches, libraries, bookstore signings, and both national and international vegetarian conferences.

You may ask, "Why leave a million dollar practice to go on the road and promote this new lifestyle?" The answer may surprise you. While researching my book, it dawned upon me that the greatest health risk of my patients was not the ear infections, colds, strep throats and allergies that so filled my daily office schedule. The real health risk for children—as well as their parents and grandparents—was a group of preventable, but fatal, chronic diseases. Heart disease, stroke, cancer and diabetes would account for the adult premature deaths of 75 percent of the children in my waiting room. The same was true of their families. And I knew that it was all basically preventable.

I learned something during the early days of the tour that would completely change the way I reached people with this new revelation, and which would set me off on a journey for which I see no ending. Though many people would read my book, something very special seemed to happen when I stood before a group of people to lecture on the life-saving benefits of proper nutrition for them and their children. Their attention seemed to be riveted on what I was saying. I felt that I was passing something on to them, over and above what they may have read in my books and essays.

I had, I told them, been holding a heavy torch—my metaphorical burden of knowledge—since the early days of my research on this subject. The only way I could carry on and lighten this increasing burden was to pass on this flame to those people attending my lectures. I would pass on to them a new responsibility that they did not have when they entered the room.

By looking into the faces of those attending my lectures, watching them nod with approval, I've been able to sustain this mounting load of evidence that our lives are increasingly at risk from a steady diet of meat and dairy products. I knew that the women and men in my audience would become a part of my journey and would share this flame with people I would never see, in places that I would never go. And in this way, I could reasonably expect to eventually reach an entire generation.

I want this book to be provocative—the best of what I've written and spoken about during this time of my life. I'm certain that you, the reader, will be surprised, sometimes shocked, and hopefully "burdened" by this new "torch of knowledge" as well, after reading these pages.

Following one of my appearances in western Canada, a ninety-five-year-old woman sent me a quote by George Bernard Shaw, the nineteenth century playwright, critic, and vegetarian. Shaw's words precisely summarize my motivation in writing this book. He says:

Life is no brief candle to me. It's a sort of splendid torch, which I've got to hold up for the moment and I want to make it burn as brightly as possible before handing it on to the next generation.

Author's Note

The following twenty-six essays, based on many of my lectures, were written during the first two years of my speaking tour. Some of the essays are modified from ideas presented in the book, *Dr. Attwood's Low-Fat Prescription for Kids* (Penguin-1995), and others from my audio series, "The Gold Standard Diet, How to Live to be 100." Other essays were published in the newsletter *New Century Nutrition*, as well as in *Nutrition Advocate*, *The European Vegetarian News* and the *American Journal of Cardiology*. These have all been updated and modified for this book. Several have appeared on my web site: www.vegsource.org/attwood, and some are published here for the first time.

I've made a strong effort in all of the essays to give the reader the facts, banish the myths, and correct the misconceptions about nutrition in America. Part One gives the simple truth we have learned from over twenty years of clinical studies, all approached from different viewpoints, but all reaching the same conclusion: that a plant-based diet is necessarily a part of the ultimate lifestyle for a long and fulfilled life. Part Two reveals some of the misinformation propagated in other publications, reveals inappropriate products and practices by the food and dairy industries, and describes the growing health hazards of certain industrial pollutants.

After most of my lectures, I've given the audience a few minutes to ask questions, which almost always introduce important and provocative ideas into the discussion. Since the reader cannot do this, some of these questions, along with my answers, are presented here, under a heading: *Ask Dr. Attwood*, following the appropriate essays.

A plant-based diet is really very simple—no calculations. The vegetables, fruits, whole grains, and legumes do it all for you. There's no need to count calories, grams of fat or protein, or worry about vitamins, minerals, antioxidants, or phytochemicals. They're all there, along with nutrients that have not yet been named, or even discovered, in the proper amounts—not too much, not too little.

When you eat more fruits and vegetables to get more beta-carotene, you not only increase your intake of the other antioxidants—C and E—you also get other protective substances that have not yet been fully studied.

—Annette B. Natow, Ph.D., R.D. Jo-Ann Heslin, M.A., R.D. *The Antioxidant Vitamin Counter*

—Charles Attwood, M.D.
April 1998

PART ONE

All You'll Ever Need to Know About the Health Risks of Food

ONE

TENDER IS THE HEART

The little girl with the long blond ponytail would have been fifty-five years old today. But there she was, on my autopsy table in 1952. The end had come suddenly and unexpectedly, from bacterial meningitis. It was my first autopsy as a medical student, and I was nervous to say the least. The professor and my fellow students were looking over my shoulder, and I was especially shaken, since this nine-year-old child had also been my "patient" a short time before.

Finally, after three tedious hours, I held her heart in my hand for a moment before beginning to open it. There, I saw, near the origin of her left anterior descending coronary, a visible yellow streak in the interior wall of the artery.

"That's cholesterol," said the professor, as he gathered the other students about me. "Look carefully, because you'll probably never see this again in a child." The fixed specimen was later added to the school's collection of medical rarities.

At that same time, unknown to all of us, autopsies were finding far greater deposits of fat in the arteries of the majority of American soldiers killed in Korea—their average age was twenty-one. Reports appeared in a major medical journal, but were largely ignored by practicing physicians. When the same findings were reported fifteen years later, during the Vietnam War, again, it was hardly noticed. Here, their Asian counterparts were also examined and found to have clean arteries.

In 1972 a twenty-five-year study began in Bogalusa, Louisiana, whereby children were examined each year. Records were made of their weights, eating habits, cholesterol levels and blood pressure; and over the years, autopsies were done on those who died accidentally. What we learned from this research shocked us all. Please sit down.

The Bogalusa Heart Study confirmed that children who eat a typical American diet have fatty deposits in their coronary arteries by age three. By age twelve, when most are entering junior high school, 70 percent have coronary fatty deposits. The deposits become much thicker and complex by the mid-teens, and virtually every adult has them by the age of twenty-one.

This largely ignored Bogalusa Heart Study was the subject of numerous conferences, two books, and over four hundred scientific articles. But the Korean, Vietnam, and Bogalusa studies, in medical libraries all over the world, gathered dust for the next several decades. No one seemed to have noticed.

These fatty deposits in children's arteries represent the early stages of coronary artery disease, but what causes them? The answer is clearly high blood-cholesterol levels, which in turn are caused by a diet too high in saturated fat and animal proteins. According to the American Heart Association, 40 million American children have abnormally high blood-cholesterol levels. This is estimated by using the federal benchmark of 170 mg/dl as the upper normal level. Most researchers now feel that this upper normal level should not exceed 150 mg/dl.

In my own pediatric practice, I find that one out of two children tested have cholesterol levels exceeding 150 mg/dl. Coronary artery disease is responsible for one-third of all adult deaths. But it doesn't appear magically at ages 40, 50, 60, or later, with the first (and often last) chest pain. It's really a childhood disease, which takes several decades to reach its endpoint. Ideally, its prevention should start during the pre-kindergarten years, by changing children's eating habits. The answer is simple: A daily diet of vegetables, fruit, whole grains and legumes. Meat, poultry, fish and dairy products should be relegated to an occasional side dish. This is the way most of the world's population eats—and they have practically no coronary disease. The "moderate" American diet is really very radical.

In the spring of 1998, the front page of every newspaper in the world ran a story about 4,000 people dying in an Afghanistan earthquake. It was big news. However, the fact that 4,000 people die every day in North America from preventable heart disease gets no attention at all. If a preventable industrial accident were killing this many people, something would be done. But for our greatest killer of all time, we simply consider it a natural part of growing old. The most vulnerable of all, now we know, are young, tender hearts.

> *Alas, regardless of their doom,*
> *the little victims play!*
> *No sense have they of ills to come*
> *Nor care beyond today.*

—Thomas Gray (1716-71)

ASK DR. ATTWOOD

Q : I'm a vegan (plant-based diet eater) and so do not have any problem insuring that I eat the World Health Organization's recommended five-to-seven helpings of fresh fruits and vegetables per day. However, I've often wondered which fruits and vegetables this is intended to include. I know, for example that potatoes are excluded. What about onions, celery, mushrooms, lettuce and cauliflower? Or does the recommendation refer only to the brightly-colored vegetables that tend to be higher in vitamins and minerals?

A : All the vegetables you mention are included. In my book, *Dr. Attwood's Low-Fat Prescription for Kids* (Penguin,1995) you will find a complete list of the most nutritious vegetables and fruits, sorted in the order of nutritional density and also in the order of consumption by Americans.

Vegetables are more nutrition dense than fruits, but the recommendation includes both. Broccoli, spinach, Brussel sprouts, lima beans, peas, asparagus, artichokes, cauliflower, sweet potatoes and carrots are near the top of the list. This information is also on my website at: http://www.vegsource.org/attwood

TWO

A WORLD EPIDEMIC GOES UNABATED

A large body of recent research evidence indicates that coronary artery disease and many types of cancer can be prevented by reducing dietary fat to approximately 10-15 percent of total calories. This is far less than the recommended guidelines (30 % of calories) issued by the American Heart Association and the National Institutes of Health.

Reducing dietary fat to 10-15 percent of calories, although not impossible for adults, is more meaningful and attainable when approached during early childhood. Eating habits, established in the preschool child, may never again be changed without severe stress. Adults, on the other hand, even after surviving a heart attack, are often unsuccessful in their attempts to significantly reduce dietary fat. Heart disease does not magically appear suddenly at ages 40, 50, or 60. This malady, the leading killer of Americans, takes twenty to forty years to develop while consuming excessive dietary fat. Since, as we have seen in the last chapter, it is already present in most young adult American men by age twenty-one, its beginnings are undoubtedly underway during the preschool years. The first symptom, often sudden death, appears much too late. So prevention should best be approached during childhood.

Some of the earliest reports by the Bogalusa Heart Study, reported in the *American Journal of Cardiology* in 1989, showed that certain children, usually white males, suddenly at puberty develop cholesterol and lipid changes, which identify them at high risk for coronary disease as early as age eleven. Again, this should indicate a need to take a look at the dietary fat of children long before these changes occur.

"In the year 2010," said Tulane pediatrician, Dr. Gerald Berenson, who founded the Bogalusa Heart Study twenty years ago, "today's children with elevated cholesterol levels will become 1.5 million heart attacks and 500,000 needless deaths unless we change their eating habits now." Dr. Berenson feels that we have ample evidence to convince anyone that this disease begins in childhood.

By the age of twelve, at least 70 percent of junior high school students in the United States already have fatty deposits in their coronary arteries. The vast majority of American soldiers killed in battle during the Korean and Vietnam wars, otherwise in good health at an average age of twenty-one, had some degree of coronary artery narrowing by cholesterol plaque.

Most other industrialized nations are experiencing the same high mortality rates from this heart disease. And again, the evidence is overwhelming that it starts very early in life. Dr. Ernst Wynder, president of the

American Health Foundation, has compared coronary deaths throughout the world with childhood cholesterol levels. "Countries with the highest death rates from coronary artery disease," he said at a recent conference, "also have the highest cholesterol levels in their children."

The same epidemic is raging in other Western nations. For instance, the fat consumption of British children has usually matched that of the United States. And in England too, adult deaths from heart disease have followed. A comparison between two British communities was reported in the *Archives of Disease of Children* by the Department of Respiratory Medicine, East Birmingham Hospital in 1990. Cholesterol levels of children were compared in these two communities that had a four-fold difference in adult mortality from coronary disease. The children from schools in the high mortality community had significantly higher cholesterol levels.

Today, however, less than 10 percent of children are being tested for their cholesterol levels by their physicians. My position, published in 1992 in *Pediatric Management* magazine, in favor of universal cholesterol testing for children, is in direct opposition to the guidelines of the American Heart Association, American Academy of Pediatrics, NIH and the AMA. They recommend that cholesterol testing should be limited to children with a family history of parents or grandparents with high cholesterol or coronary heart disease. The enormous expense cited by these agencies (a cholesterol test on a child costs the physician about $2.50) pales when compared to the cost of this disease, once it has developed, including direct medical expenses, absenteeism, insurance and job retraining—estimated at $200 billion annually in the U.S.

Good Study, but Wrong Conclusion

A study in Muscatine, Iowa in 1990, conducted by the University of Iowa, has been quoted by the National Institutes of Health and the American Academy of Pediatrics as showing a poor relationship between children's high cholesterol levels to high levels later as adults. I reviewed this study very carefully and came to an entirely different conclusion. During a fifteen-year follow-up of 2367 children, 70 percent who had cholesterol levels exceeding the 90th percentile, later had adult levels that are considered high according to the present guidelines of the NIH's National Cholesterol Education Program.

Undoubtedly, the American Academy of Pediatrics and the NIH have misinterpreted the Muscatine, Iowa studies and issued misleading guidelines affecting at least one third of the nation's children who may be at risk and never know it until the disease strikes them later as adults.

As for using family history as a criterion for cholesterol screening in children, this is nonsense. I've insisted in my essays and seminars that parents of most children are still too young to have had *symptoms* of coronary heart disease. Dr. Richard E. Garcia, co-director of the pediatric lipid clinic at the Cleveland Clinic foundation did cholesterol levels on 6500 children. Families of 299 of the 375 with high cholesterol levels were contacted. Nearly half (48 percent) reported no history of cholesterol problems or heart disease in siblings, parents, grandparents, aunts or uncles. By following the NIH guidelines, at least half would never have had a cholesterol determination during their entire childhood.

In another report by the Department of Pediatrics of Chicago's Northwestern University Medical School, published in *Pediatrics* in 1989, family history factors recommended by the NIH and AAP as criteria for cholesterol screening in children *did not* identify half of all the children found to have abnormally high cholesterol levels. The study concluded that in order to find the children with abnormally high cholesterol levels, *all* children must be tested at least once.

In a 1992 study of 650 northern Italian children, elevated levels of cholesterol were found to be correlated only with the intake of fat. The study concluded that a family history of cardiovascular disease did not identify the children at risk.

Data from a 1989 health census in Otsego County, N.Y., showed that in 16 percent of the population, family health information was either unavailable or unknown for one of the parents. This rate reflects the findings of national studies, according to Dr. Barbara Dennison of the Mary Imogene Bassett Hospital, Cooperstown, N.Y. So, once again, family history is an unreliable criteria for checking children's levels.

The Bent Twig Effect

It's much easier to establish a low fat, plant-based diet during early childhood than having to adopt one later after coronary disease is already established. Dietary habits that are well established by age 8-10 will likely last a lifetime.

Approximately 40 percent of the 6000 children recently tested in my clinic have cholesterol levels above 170 mg/dl. One might expect that the parents of these children would dismiss this as nothing more ominous than a little extra weight. Not so. I've been amazed by the response of parents as I talk about a plant-based diet for reducing their child's intake of saturated fat. Almost always, when the child's cholesterol level is rechecked three months later, it is reduced significantly.

Unfortunately, coronary artery disease has become accepted as an inevitable part of our culture. Therefore, most of the NIH and private foundation funds have been committed to high-tech treatment and rehabilitation, with only token spending on prevention. Only one-tenth as many deaths each year result from automobile accidents, yet the manufacturers and federal government have spent far more in an effort to prevent them.

A Dietary Hazard: Milk and Dairy Products

The most damaging source of saturated fat available to children is undoubtedly milk and dairy products. In October, 1992, the Physicians Committee for Responsible Medicine (PCRM), headed by Dr. Neal Barnard, held a Washington, DC press conference, where the late Dr. Frank Osiki, of Johns Hopkins and other nutrition experts spoke out against all consumption of cow's milk during infancy and childhood. They cited the growing evidence of life-long allergies, coronary heart disease, cancer, and even insulin-dependent diabetes.

Suzanne Havala, a registered dietitian from North Carolina, who was a co-author of the American Dietetic Association's 1992 edition of its position paper on vegetarian diets stated at the Washington press conference that, after weaning, there is no need for milk of any sort. "Vegetarians and their children," she said, "get all the calcium they need from leafy vegetables, broccoli, tahini and tofu made with calcium sulfate."

Dr. Russell J. Bunai, a pediatrician associated with the PCRM, who later took a two-year sabbatical from his practice to review the world literature on the subject, said, " . . . of all mammals, only humans drink the milk of another species." In Ghana, where he served as a medical missionary, he noted that the traditional diet contains no dairy products and that asthma and other allergic problems were uncommon. He saw these problems only in people who had adopted more westernized diets that included cow's milk. Here, we should add that coronary artery disease is rarely seen in Ghana among those who consume only this traditional diet.

Not unexpectedly, the American Academy of Pediatrics issued an immediate rebuttal through Harvard professor Dr. Ronald E. Kleinman, chairman of the AAP's committee on nutrition. He said that pediatricians should trust the advice they have been giving for the last one hundred years. "Pediatricians should recognize that this group is practicing 'nutritional terrorism,'" he added. I responded with a personal message reminding him that during the last hundred years, coronary artery disease has become our number-one killer, whereas, before the turn of the century, it wasn't among the top ten causes of death.

I strongly agree with the PCRM position. It's a necessary first step in reducing total fat, and especially saturated fat, in the diets of children. During my forty-year practice, as a board-certified pediatrician, I've observed the damaging effects of cow's milk in eight out of every ten children I see. Milk first sensitizes the child to later allergic disorders, and it's the single largest source of cholesterol-raising saturated fat. Eliminating cow's milk is necessarily the hallmark of any meaningful program for reducing dietary fat in children to 10-15 percent of calories, and preventing coronary artery disease.

According to an overly optimistic statement made in 1994 by Dr. Paul Savello, a professor at Utah State University, "In five years there will be no more whole milk for sale in grocery stores." He added that in fifteen to twenty years, 2 percent milk would also disappear from the supermarket shelves. Actually 2 percent milk, then allowed by the FDA to be labeled as "low fat," derives nearly 37 percent of its calories from fat, most of which are saturated. After 1998, 2 percent milk must be labeled "reduced fat." Hopefully, this too will disappear from the grocery shelves much sooner than Dr. Savello had predicted.

The True Risk of Obesity

Dietary fat during childhood may be more life threatening than was originally suspected. A 1992 study by Dr. Aviva Must, an epidemiologist at the United States department of Agriculture's Human Nutrition Research Center at Tufts University in Boston, revealed that adolescent obesity in males is associated with a much higher death rate (double) from heart attacks, strokes, and colon cancer by age seventy than in adolescents of normal weight. This was true even in cases where the youngsters later shed the excess weight. The death rates were also much higher than when obesity had its onset later during adulthood.

The obvious conclusion was that an early childhood intervention is best. But unfortunately, children's weights are on the increase. A Center for Disease Control and Prevention (CDC) report in 1995 revealed that one in five U.S. children (ages 6-17) is overweight and the percentage of children who are the most severely obese has doubled since 1960.

The Epidemic is Global

No better model exists of the adult effects of children's dietary fat than that of the Japanese, who have historically raised their children on diets consisting of less than 10 percent fat calories. Accordingly, Japan is among the nations of the world with the lowest incidence of coronary disease in adults. Furthermore, life expectancy in Japan leads all other nations where records are available. Unfortunately, this sparkling example may not continue.

In most urban areas the Japanese diet has become Americanized. The levels of fat intake since World War II have been steadily increasing. While total calories have not changed, daily fat intake was 16 grams in 1946, 27.8 grams in 1961, and 56.8 grams in 1985. Therefore dietary fat has doubled during the last twenty-five years and nearly tripled during the post war period. During this same time, studies by the Department of Pathology at

Kyushu University in Fukuoka has shown that coronary deaths have been increasing over the last forty years, but are still less than those found in autopsy cases in Boston.

In a nationwide cooperative study of atherosclerosis in young Japanese, atherosclerotic changes were observed to begin developing during childhood. And once again, serum cholesterol levels were strongly correlated with the extent of fatty streaks in the coronary arteries. The authors of the report, published in *Atherosclerosis* in 1988, concluded that primary prevention of atherosclerosis should be initiated in the pediatric age group.

Coronary disease has also increased among adults in other countries following several decades of Americanized diets for their children. China, France and Italy are the most recent examples, where children's dietary fat is increasing in urban areas to levels common to the United States. Whole populations are shifting from diseases of poverty to diseases of affluence. No government health agency seems ready to address the problem as we approach the twenty-first century.

A report in the *International Journal of Cardiology* in 1990 described autopsy studies of one hundred children in the Italian region of Veneto who had died from causes unrelated to the cardiovascular system. The children of northern Italy in general have had increased dietary fat and higher cholesterol for several decades. Thickenings were found in the left anterior-descending coronary artery in 95.3 percent of the age group between one and five years. Actual mature fibrous plaques were found in fifteen children. The authors of the report expressed concern because of recent reports of sudden coronary deaths in young people from the same geographic area.

Hong Kong, Taiwan and Mainland China have all had increasing levels of fat in their children's diets since the 1950s. These three areas still have much less coronary disease—about one-fourth to one-eighth that of the United States—than most western countries. However, according to a study by the Chinese University of Hong Kong in 1989, while coronary disease is now decreasing in the West, these three areas, with a population of 1.2 billion, is experiencing a sharp increase in the disease.

It's even worse when we focus on large cities. Mortality rates from coronary heart disease in Singapore have reached levels comparable with the United States. According to the Department of Community, Occupational, and Family Medicine at the National University Hospital in Singapore, levels of dietary fat and cholesterol levels have reached levels similar to Western countries.

These studies in our own country and throughout the world should give our Federal Government and organized scientific groups a clear mandate to recommend further meaningful reductions in dietary fat for both children and adults. Their guidelines, however, appear to be fixed, without signs of change in the foreseeable future.

ASK DR. ATTWOOD

Q: I am a vegetarian living in Seoul, Korea. I'm concerned about the level of pollution in this city. Are there any dietary or supplemental choices that I could make to help combat the effects of living in a polluted environment?

A: Environmental pollution is also a concern to us here in the United States. A plant–based diet, without supplements, and pure water is very important. If you are also worried about pesticide residues on your vegetables and fruits, peel or wash them. Generally, the benefits of eating vegetables and fruits far outweigh any negative effects from pesticide residues. Of course, organically grown food would be best, when available. The only thing you can't control is the air you breathe. But let's face it, the greatest pollutant is animal fat and protein. Avoid that and you will overcome the less serious effects of air pollution.

THREE

A VEGETARIAN CLAN

Dr. Caldwell B. Esselstyn, Jr., a thyroid surgeon at the Cleveland Clinic, had long questioned the traditional treatment approach to coronary artery disease. This leading killer of Americans, he observed, must be prevented rather than treated by surgery and high-tech coronary care. "It's the result," he told his colleagues," of too much saturated fat, usually beginning during childhood." Quoting the late Dr. Denis Burkitt, famed proponent of dietary fiber, he metaphorically suggested a different plan of attack on this leading killer:

> If people are falling over the edge of a cliff and sustaining injuries, the problem could be dealt with by stationing ambulances at the bottom or erecting a fence at the top. Unfortunately, we put far too much effort into positioning of ambulances and far too little into the simple approach of erecting fences.

Dr. Esselstyn's idea: Why not conduct "A Summit Meeting" of the nation's top nutritional scientists willing to speak out on new research data that most doctors and government agencies have been reluctant to recommend? Such a meeting would bring together the top researchers in nutrition and coronary artery disease to share their latest findings with practicing physicians who were interested in preventing coronary disease. Then, hopefully, the truth would "trickle down" to parents, physicians and educators.

A Summit Meeting was an ambitious project, but finally, in October 1991, under the sponsorship of the Caldwell B. Esselstyn Foundation and the Cleveland Clinic Foundation, the First National Conference on the Elimination of Coronary Artery Disease was held at Loew's Ventana Canyon Resort, outside Tucson, Arizona. For two days, thirteen leading scientists discussed their research projects. Along with fifty practicing physicians from almost every area of the country, I attended as a physician-journalist for thirty Louisiana newspapers.

For two days everyone sat with their attention riveted on speaker after speaker from 8:00 A.M. to 5:00 A.M., while vacationers at the resort, surrounded by tall, flowering cacti (some towering fifty feet), played golf and tennis. Over coffee and snacks at every break, discussions continued in small clusters.

According to the hotel restaurants there were more requests for vegetarian meals than at any other time in its history. Anticipating this, Dr. Esselstyn arranged for Mr. Roy Guste, former owner of Antoine's Restaurant in New Orleans and author of the new cookbook, *Louisiana Light*, to prepare a lowfat, but tasty lunch on the first day of the conference.

Incredibly, researchers who had taken entirely different approaches, all reached the same conclusion: Not only is the typical American diet much too high in fat, protein and calories, but the guidelines of the American Heart Association, recommending no more than 30 percent of calories from fat, is not nearly low enough. Also, the shocker: Their studies reported an actual progression of existing coronary disease on this officially recommended diet.

The participants in this historic meeting affirmed what we've stressed throughout this book. The ideal diet, according to most of the experts, is plant-based, with little or no animal products, deriving only 10-15 percent of its calories from fat. The ideal time to start such a diet is during childhood before a taste for fat is fully developed.

The famed China Study was explained by its director, Cornell's Dr. T. Colin Campbell. Coronary disease was almost unknown in villages consuming an all-plant diet and it was common in villages where meat and dairy products were eaten.

"But what about us Americans who already have this disease?" someone asked. It was common knowledge that most of us in the conference had varying degrees of coronary disease already—along with an estimated 60-80 million other adults in this country. Since we didn't prevent it during our youth, what were we to do now?

"It's never too late," commented Dr. Dean Ornish. A vegetarian diet, without animal products can actually *reverse* coronary artery disease, without bypass surgery. Interestingly, the *control* subjects in the Ornish studies were on the American Heart Asssociation diet guideline (no more than 30 percent of calories from fat), and they had *progression* of their coronary plaques.

Everyone at the conference agreed that coronary disease begins several decades before its first symptom—which may be sudden death. Dr. Gerald Berenson of Louisiana State University, director of the Bogulosa Heart Study, which was then already in its nineteenth year, presented his data, proving that coronary heart disease starts in early childhood. He and the other researchers on the panel recommended that children over age two should be on the same vegetarian-type diet as adults.

During the first morning session, the thirteen scientists were asked by Dr. Ernst Wynder to make a strong public statement relating the consumption of saturated fat to coronary heart disease and the obvious relationship between smoking and lung cancer. Being another strong advocate of reducing dietary fat in children, he reminded us of the findings of a world survey conducted by his own American Health Foundation—that throughout the world, wherever the adult death rate from coronary disease is high, the cholesterol levels of that nation's children are high.

As we all expected, dairy products didn't fare well at the conference. The general consensus among practicing pediatricians at the time was to recommend low-fat milk for all children over the age of two. But, Dr. Campbell pointed out that low-fat (2 percent) milk isn't actually low-fat at all—thirty-six percent of its calories are from fat, most of which is saturated. As we have noted earlier, this wasn't significantly less than the fat in whole milk (50 percent of calories), even through federal regulations at the time allowed it to be labeled "low-fat," and this regulation changed in 1998, after which 2 percent milk was required to be labeled "reduced fat." My *Four Stages to an Ideal Diet*, which was not to be published for another four years, recommended no milk or other dairy products at all.

Framingham Study director, Dr. William Castelli, told the group that coronary heart disease is extremely rare in the three-fourths of the world's population who do *not* consume our Western high-fat, high-protein diet. The rural Chinese, he said, have very low cholesterol levels of about 100-120 mg/dl and almost no coronary disease, although the great majority of men smoke cigarettes.

"There's never been a heart attack death reported with a total cholesterol under 150 in the forty-year history of the Framingham Study," said Dr. Castelli.

"And this takes a lot more dietary restraint than simply avoiding red meat and removing skin from chicken and turkey," commented director and moderator Dr. Caldwell Esselstyn from his seat near the podium, where he remained throughout the meeting.

Dr. Ronald Hart, director of the National Center of Toxicological Research and Cornell's Dr. Colin Campbell described their independent studies on mice. Caloric restriction of Dr. Hart's mice was associated with a reduction of tumors and greater longevity. The mice lived 50 percent longer and, surprisingly, just died suddenly without disease.

Dr. Campbell's mice showed the same reduction of tumors and increased life span when fed a diet with greatly reduced animal protein. The young mice in both studies had less dietary fat than the controls.

Toward the end of the second day it was clear that no

one in the great meeting room—neither the panelists (with the exception of two employees of the NIH) nor the fifty physicians in attendance—believed that the current American Heart Association guidelines were low enough. Then, as if to give this opinion a final and poetic tribute, as the conference was in its final hour, Dr. Campbell walked to the podium and eloquently summarized what was to be our consensus.

> If we are all sure of what our data from these studies is telling us, then why must we be reticent about recommending a diet which we know is safe and healthy? We, as scientists, can no longer take the attitude that the public cannot benefit from information they are not ready for.
>
> We must have the integrity to tell them the truth and let them decide what to do with it. We cannot force them to follow the guidelines we recommend, but we can give them these guidelines and then let the public decide. I personally have great faith in the public.
>
> We must tell them that a diet of roots, stems, seeds, flowers, fruit, and leaves is the healthiest diet and the only diet we can promote, endorse, and recommend.

As he walked back to his seat, everyone in the room applauded. Dr. Ornish agreed: "Most physicians are underestimating the ability of the people to accept our scientific findings." He said that we shouldn't be giving advice based on what we think will be accepted, but rather on what we have found that "works."

The conference ended, and we said goodbye. Dr. Esselstyn, now in jeans and a straw hat, joined a group of us for a visit to nearby Biosphere 2. Tall, slender and athletic, this 1956 Olympic Gold Medallist had found new hope in his "Summit in the Desert." "It's possible," he said, "that people someday in the not-too-distant future, like Dr. Hart's mice, will live a great deal longer and just die suddenly of old age—without disease."

This conference was repeated in September 1997, sponsored and developed by the Cleveland Clinic and hosted by the Walt Disney company at the Disney Institute in Orlando, Florida. It was attended by five hundred doctors and healthcare professionals, ten times the attendance at the first conference. At the Disney conference I was a member of the faculty and my lecture appears in the 1998 issue of the *American Journal of Cardiology.*

ASK DR. ATTWOOD

Q: I tried vegetarianism for four months and never was I more tired or miserable. I felt good the first thirty days, and after that I could not get enough protein out of the vegetables.

A: Your problem is likely too much protein, not too little. Many studies document the onset of coronary heart disease or progression on existing heart disease on 30 percent fat calories. This does not happen with 20 percent or lower, which requires a vegetarian diet. The diet most people already eat has led to the greatest epidemic of coronary heart disease in world history.

FOUR

A BREASTFEEDING STORY

There's one type of food everyone should have consumed at one time in his or her life. It isn't plant-based. It isn't low-fat. But its effect on our ultimate health is enormous. Unfortunately, some people never get it—it's breastmilk.

Breastmilk is available to every infant. It's free. It's clean. It's the right temperature, and it's convenient. It also, according to one of my medical school professors, comes in cute containers.

My great, great, great grandfather, Dr. Curtis Burke Attwood, who practiced medicine in Newberry, South Carolina during the late 1700s, wouldn't have believed that we have people today who specialize as breastfeeding consultants. They are certified by their own board, the International Board of Lactation Consultant Examiners. In my grandfather's day, practically all women breast-fed their babies, but today only 59.7 percent start breastfeeding in the hospital, and after six months all but 21.6 percent have given up. The Healthy

People 2000 breastfeeding objective is to have 75 percent of women leave the hospital breastfeeding and 50 percent continuing to do so six months later. Obviously, we're falling far short of this goal.

The advantages of breastfeeding are enormous. Babies have less acute illnesses and allergies. The bonding between the mother and her baby is enhanced far beyond that between mothers and bottle-fed babies. So why are only one-fifth of six-month-olds still breastfeeding?

I've always complained to my colleagues that we don't take enough time to explain these procedures and other good health practices to our patients. Usually, this means we don't give them time to ask questions. But, these days, new mothers barely spend twenty-four hours in the hospital, so we may not have the opportunity to explain things adequately—and often they don't ask. It's no wonder we think we're misunderstood. I had a patient recently, who, although intimidated by our busy, distant manner, desperately needed some basic information. She tried.

Gloria, the young mother, had just given birth to her first child at my hospital. She called the nursery and asked if she could still breast-feed the baby, even though she had a cold. "I'm sneezing and coughing," she said, "and I'm worried." She was going home that same day and she wanted some answers.

Pleased that she had chosen to breast-feed, I told the nurse to tell her to go ahead. I suggested that the nurse leave a couple of facemasks on her bedside table. That way Gloria wouldn't worry so much. We should have personally talked to her about breastfeeding, but she was being discharged and there wasn't much time.

Later, during rounds, I dropped by her room. "Hello, Gloria," I said as I sauntered into the room, and then I saw something that I'll never forget as long as I live. Now, put yourself in my place. I could hardly retreat from the room with a straight face. I found Gloria with a confused expression on her face and a facemask on each breast.

After the story was repeated throughout the hospital and the laughter finally died down in the doctor's lounge, I thought of Gloria's humiliation and her sincere need for the information we didn't have time to give her. Grandfather Curtis Burke Attwood wouldn't have thought it was so funny.

ASK DR. ATTWOOD

Q: I breast-fed my baby for six months before I returned to work. Since I started her on a regular cow's milk formula, she has a dry scaly rash on her face and neck. My pediatrician calls it eczema and says, "Don't worry about it." The baby also has frequent loose bowel movements and cramping. Would you recommend that soy milk substitute be used? And if so, is there any reason to worry about a baby who may never be able to drink cow's milk?

A: Your dilemma is shared by millions of working mothers in this country. The fact that you have continued to breast-feed for six months is commendable. Whenever infants are unable to continue breastfeeding and have been found to be intolerant to cow's milk—or actually allergic to the cow's milk protein—I reluctantly recommend a commercial soy formula until such time as the child is eating an adequate solid diet.

Ideally, a mother should breast-feed up to two years if possible. By six months of age most infants can eat soft solids (prepared with a blender) from the family table food. The majority of infants seem to tolerate commercial soy formulas very well.

So why am I cautious? It's possible that early exposure to soy proteins through daily use of commercial soy formulas may sensitize babies to soy allergies later in life, just as the early exposure to cow's milk can lead to milk allergies such as eczema, asthma and rhinitis.

FIVE

THE "COMPLETE PROTEIN" MYTH

It's Time to Set the Record Straight

Nothing has given vegetarianism a worse reputation than the "Complete Protein Myth." Meat and dairy products were thought to be necessary in order to obtain all of the amino acids required to build protein. The time has come to finally dispel one of the last great misconceptions of clinical nutrition. Not surprisingly, this myth has persisted largely because of misinformation trumpeted for decades by the beef and dairy industries.

In the 1971 first edition of *Diet for a Small Planet* by Francis Moore Lappé, she suggested that vegetables be combined carefully with legumes or soybeans to insure a supply of essential amino acids, important components of these so-called "complete proteins." Later however, in the 1991 edition of the book, she reassured her readers that this was "a myth," and that any reasonable variety of vegetables would suffice. Unfortunately, the attention this particular subject received in the first edition was essentially overlooked in the last edition. Vegetarianism has therefore been unpopular to millions, regardless of its health benefits, because they considered it to be too complex and cumbersome. It's time to set the record straight.

Proteins are composed of amino acids, twelve of which are manufactured by the human body. Another nine, known as essential amino acids, must be obtained from food. Most animal foods, such as meat and dairy products, contain all of the essential amino acids, and have therefore been designated as containing *complete* proteins. This is misleading because most proteins from vegetables also contain all essential amino acids.

Now here's the part that's *really* misunderstood. The proteins we eat are not used as such. They are broken down into these amino acids, joined by the amino acids produced by the body and even more amino acids from the metabolic breakdown of tissue proteins—a process known as catabolism. From this enormous pool of amino acids, new specific proteins are built for use throughout the body.

So it makes no difference where these amino acids come from, whether they are from plant or animal sources. Thus, the old myth that vegetarians must carefully *combine* foods to insure "complete proteins" makes no sense. Practically, *any* variety of vegetables supplies adequate amounts of essential amino acids. There will be no protein deficiency from a plant-based diet as long as enough calories are consumed.

It *does* make a difference, however, whether or not these sources are excessive—as they usually are when obtained from animal sources. In America and other Western nations, over two-thirds of proteins are obtained from meat and dairy products. Their protein consumption, therefore, is excessive, often 100-120 grams daily, when the proper amount for most adults is 50-60 grams. Meat and dairy consumers are overburdened with protein, which has been related to a variety of serious disorders, such as kidney disease, heart disease, cancer and osteoporosis. These diseases are almost unknown in two-thirds of the world population, including the rural Chinese and Japanese, who get 90 percent of their protein from vegetable sources.

ASK DR. ATTWOOD

Q: Although I am a vegetarian, I am concerned, that I'm not getting enough protein in my diet. Currently I derive most of my protein from dairy products such as cottage cheese, yogurt and other milk products, and beans. Are there other suggestions you would make for me to insure I get enough protein?

A: Let me reassure you, there's plenty of quality protein in a vegetarian diet—even without the dairy products. A reasonable variety of vegetables, grains and legumes will supply all essential amino acids.

SIX

MEAT-EATERS ARE MADE, NOT BORN.

The fact that one's taste for meat and dairy products is not a part of the human genetic blueprint often comes as a surprise to families coming to my clinic. Virginia, the mother of two teenage boys, appeared in my office in a state of confusion. Typical of many parents I see, she felt that her family's taste for meat, high-fat dairy products and pastries was inborn and, therefore, a lifelong burden.

"I thought it was natural," Virginia told me. "It seems like all the boys' friends stuff themselves on pizza, hamburgers and french fries." Then, shaking her head, she added, "Besides, my husband would die without *his* steak and fried chicken!"

Like many other wives and mothers, Virginia assumed that trying to change her family's eating habits would be futile. Not so! I explained to her that her husband and children had each acquired a desire for meat and other animal products when they were quite young; they weren't born with it. No matter how closely you examine the human tongue, no taste buds for fat can be found—there are only sweet, sour, salty and bitter sensors.

The desire for fat is learned, and it results from a combination of the way these foods smell, and their smoothness on the mouth's surface. Butter and ice cream, for example, are said to "melt" in one's mouth. Often used to sell products, fat is frequently combined with refined sugars in a single product to make it more "palatable." This combination is found in desserts, pastries, candy, cookies and almost all packaged snacks—all high in fat, though commonly referred to as "sweets." In essence, the fat taste is just a habit created by conditioning.

All too often, high-fat foods, or "sweets," are held out as rewards to children for "good" behavior. Dr. Leann Birch, at the University of Illinois Child Development Laboratory, has found that in Western countries young children are conditioned or taught to like animal-based foods. For example, how many times have you heard parents say, "You can have your ice cream if you eat your spinach"? Children then quickly assume that if ice cream is the reward, then spinach must be the punishment. By contrast, most children in rural China and Japan, who haven't been offered such a deal, are repulsed by the thought of eating animals or the foods made from them.

Still, my patient Virginia wasn't entirely convinced. She had two sons, ages fourteen and seventeen. "If the fat taste is already thoroughly ingrained," she asked, "what can I possibly do about my teenagers?" Good question. I went on to explain that older children, and even adults, are not destined to live out the rest of their lives with an addiction to meat and dairy products acquired during their youth. During my thirty-five years of clinical practice, I've seen many parents, and even grandparents, of my young patients change to a plant-based diet. Often this has resulted after I've found a high cholesterol level in one of the children and then discovered that this was part of a family pattern.

Clinical studies seem to confirm the experiences in my clinic—the taste for fat and animal products can readily be changed. Dr. Richard Mattes, a researcher at the Monell Chemical Senses Center in Philadelphia, reported in 1993 that when fatty foods were sharply reduced or eaten only rarely, the desire for them declined, or even disappeared entirely, after eight to twelve weeks. One warning, however. He also found that if moderate amounts of high-fat foods were continued, whether as side dishes or condiments, the fat taste persisted.

Further clinical evidence comes from the Fred Hutchinson Cancer Research Center in Seattle, which surveyed 448 women participants in a program to reduce dietary fat. A majority of the women said that while they were on the program, which lasted for several weeks, they lost their taste for fat. Returning to fatty foods after the program ended resulted in a variety of gastrointestinal complaints—cramping, bloating—for most, whether or not they had lost their taste for fat.

Virginia and her family were given my *Four Stages to an Ideal Diet* (see page 107) to use as a guide when food-shopping and cooking. I assured Virginia that once the family reached Stage Three—consisting of vegetables, fruits, whole grains and legumes, with only occasional consumption of meat and dairy products—they would be well on their way toward taming their fat tastes. And, by the time they arrived at Stage Four (with no meat or dairy products), they'd have banished the fat taste completely.

Hopefully, Virginia's grandchildren will not need these transitions. I've seen Stage Four toddlers who never had to bother with Stages One through Three! Whereas children and healthy adults seem to need these gradual diet changes, adults with heart disease, stroke or other fat-related disorders, may successfully go directly to Stage Four.

Dr. Dean Ornish has found that a totally plant-based diet is less difficult for his patients to attain when it's done suddenly, without first trying moderate reductions in fat. They have the added assurance of the diet's positive health gains—lower cholesterol levels, weight loss, and a vastly reduced risk of death from heart disease and cancer—not fully attainable while still eating even modest amounts of fat.

Following a mild stroke, my good friend, the late Dr. Spock, made the switch at age eighty-eight. He resumed writing, lecturing and traveling until his death on March 15, 1998 at the age of ninety-four.

ASK DR. ATTWOOD

Q: Some of my friends insist that they experience weakness and lose stamina without meat in their diet. I've worried about this as I continue to cut down on all animal products. Will I eventually find that my exercise program, mostly jogging and walking, will be compromised?

A: I'm virtually certain that you can enjoy the best of both—a plant-based diet and aerobic exercise. Some of the best athletes I've known, including marathoners and body builders are vegans. As for myself, I've remained physically active since I became a vegetarian fifteen years ago. I've never felt better. I strongly suspect the weakness perceived by some who discontinue meat is the result of a lifetime of "brain washing" by the meat industry.

SEVEN

MILK, A CATCH-22

Calcium Without the Cow

The young mother of a seven-year-old boy handed me a note from the grade-school dietitian. "Billy's diet has come to our attention," it read, "because he no longer selects milk in the cafeteria." Billy had recently given up milk, at my suggestion, because it worsened his asthma and eczema. The note concluded, "Milk is absolutely necessary for protein and calcium!" and this last sentence was heavily underlined. I quickly realized how concerned Billy's mother was. Besides the dietitian's warning, she was also dealing with the fact that several elderly members of her family had a history of osteoporosis—a condition for which dairy products are highly recommended.

This same dilemma is encountered most frequently by families who are trying to reduce saturated fat and animal protein in their diets. They've read that both may increase the risk of heart disease and certain cancers, but worry about calcium balance and bone density if milk, the chief source of saturated fat for children, is discontinued. I often reassure concerned parents that some

45

bowing of their child's legs is normal up to the age of three, and is not due to a calcium deficiency or rickets. Dental decay in early childhood causes the same concern, but ironically it is partially due to the frequent bathing of the teeth with milk, rather than a calcium deficiency.

Why is this paranoia so common among Americans? The milk-calcium-bone-density myth has been created and perpetuated by the intense lobbying of the dairy industry throughout the lifetimes of most adults living today. Throughout kindergarten and grade school, most of the nutrition-teaching aids were supplied by the American Dairy Council. As a result, most parents, teachers, doctors, lawyers, judges and, significantly, members of Congress grew up with the not unbiased view that milk is a necessary and wholesome food for both children and adults. The Dairy Council's most effective campaign tool has been to link milk, calcium and bone density.

To further confuse the consumer, milk and infant formulas have been fortified with vitamin D, which is necessary for proper calcium absorption. It may also be obtained by eating sardines, herring, salmon, tuna, egg yolk or fish oils. However, none of these are necessary, because vitamin D is manufactured in adequate amounts by exposure to as little as ten to fifteen minutes of sunlight about three times a week. Rickets may be prevented in children who get no sunlight—such as the severely disabled—by a vitamin D supplement, if the parents do not wish to feed them fortified milk.

The true connection between milk and strong bones isn't exactly what the dairy industry has been telling us all these years. Calcium balance—the relationship between the intake and loss of the mineral—determines bone density mostly during childhood and adolescence. Good bone density attained by the age of eighteen usually lasts a lifetime for people who consume a balanced plant-based diet and remain physically active. Milk and other dairy products, although rich in calcium, are high in animal protein, which has been shown to create calcium loss through the urinary tract.

A 1994 National Institute of Health Consensus Conference concluded that calcium balance and bone density depended, at least 30 percent, on the ratio of intake to loss, not on calcium intake alone. According to a report in *Science* magazine in 1986, evidence is accumulating that calcium intake (considered alone) is not related to bone density. This may explain why countries consuming the most milk also have the highest incidence of osteoporosis. Exceptions exist, but a common determining factor seems to be the high-protein consumption in populations who require very high levels of calcium intake. For instance, the RDA of calcium in the United States is up to 1,200 mg. daily. This is much higher than the World Health Organization's recommendation of 500 mg. for children and 800 mg. for adults. Areas of the world where dietary protein is very low have low national recommendations. In Thailand, for example, the recommended daily intake of calcium is only 400 mg. for all ages. Elderly South African Bantu women, who consume a very low protein diet (50 grams daily, compared with 91 grams for Americans) and only 450 mg. of calcium daily, have no osteoporosis despite the calcium drain of nursing an average of ten children. On the other hand, Eskimos, who consume a very high protein diet (250-400 grams) of fish, and have a calcium intake of over 2,000 mg. daily, have the highest rate of osteoporosis in the world!

Now let's take a new look at milk and dairy products as a calcium source, regardless of their protein content. When calcium is expressed in mg. per 100 calories (instead of per gram), milk and cheese fall at the bottom of the list, and green vegetables appear at the top:

Calcium in Milligrams per 100 Calories

Arugula	1,300
Watercress	800
Turnip greens	650
Collard greens	548
Mustard greens	490
Spinach	450
Broccoli	387
Swiss cheese	250
Milk (2-percent)	245
Green onions	240
Okra	213
Cabbage	196
Whole milk	190
Cheddar cheese	179
American cheese	160

At first glance one may conclude: "But I would have to eat so much more spinach or kale to get adequate calcium." Not so. Individuals on a plant-based diet generally eat as many total calories as meat and dairy-eaters. In other words, adequate amounts of vegetables are *better sources of calcium than milk and cheese.* Also, consider that a cup of broccoli contains about the same amount of calcium as a cup of milk. But wait! Haven't we been told that many green vegetables contain oxalic acid, which reduces the absorption of their calcium. This too, has been exaggerated by the dairy lobby. A 1990 report in the *American Journal of Clinical Nutrition* concluded that greens such as broccoli and kale have high levels of calcium that are absorbed at least as well as that in milk. Excellent calcium balance on a non-dairy diet is easily attained because ALL vegetables and legumes contain calcium, and collectively it's more than adequate. This calcium stays in the bones, unlike much of that from the high protein-containing dairy products.

Now it all begins to make sense. In cultures where the most protein is consumed, the calcium requirement for good bone density and protection against osteoporosis may be *unattainably* high without supplements—it's a Catch-22. But for the majority of the world population, and among those consuming a plant-based diet in Western countries, calcium requirements for normal bone density are easily obtained without milk or other dairy products. Milk, it now seems clear, is not the solution to the malady of poor bone density. In fact, milk may be a part of the problem! You *can* have your calcium without the cow.

ASK DR. ATTWOOD

Q: My mother just fractured her hip. According to her doctor, the fracture was caused by severe osteoporosis. She drank milk daily since childhood and ate cheese with most meals. She also ate meat daily, including beef, poultry and fish. I'm concerned about the prospects of my own family. We eat very little meat or dairy products. We eat lots of fresh vegetables and fruits. We don't drink milk as a beverage, but do add skim milk to our breakfast cereals. I've heard that the protein in milk can promote calcium loss. Should we worry about the small amount of skim milk we are using?

A: I share your concern about osteoporosis. At my age, it seems that more and more friends and acquaintances have brittle bones. Like your mother, most of them consumed milk and other dairy products—as well as meat—daily throughout their lives.

You are to be complimented on what appears to be an excellent diet to protect your family from this terrible malady in their later years. It's true that excessive protein in the diet, especially from animal sources, tends to promote calcium loss—even as it is being consumed in the form of dairy products. The acidification of the blood by protein causes the kidneys to excrete calcium. A diet of vegetables, fruits, whole grains and legumes supplies adequate calcium, without excessive protein.

The thing to remember here is that vegetarians maintain their bone density without dairy products, and the disease is commonly found, like in your mother's case, among people who consume milk and dairy products throughout their lives. Since the overall protein-intake in your family's diet is not excessive, I would not worry about any calcium-losing effect of the small amount of skim milk in the breakfast cereal. Ideally, however, I like to avoid all animal protein. Your skim milk could be replaced by rice or soy milk.

❦❦❦

Q: I've heard that some of us, as we grow older, run the risk of deficiencies in vitamin D. What causes this, and how can we prevent it?

A: There may be some impairment of vitamin D metabolism as one ages, but my opinion is that many elderly people get inadequate sunlight. This is especially true among the disabled. Throughout most of our lives, adequate vitamin D is manufactured by exposure to the sun, a minimum of ten-to-fifteen minutes of sunlight three times a week.

If this isn't possible, a vitamin D supplement or fortified food is recommended. I should also point out that excessive direct sunlight exposure to the skin might lead to skin cancer. For this reason, I wear a straw hat with a wide brim.

EIGHT

MOTHER NATURE'S WAY

A Woman's Greatest Health Risk

When the chest pains started, Mary was on her regular flight from Miami to San Francisco. At age forty-six, she had worked as a flight attendant on American Airlines for over twenty years without missing a single day due to illness. Mary had always enjoyed excellent health—or so she thought. Now, within three hours she would find herself in a coronary care unit, where she would be told that three coronary vessels were partially occluded, but one, the left anterior-descending, was 95 percent blocked.

A balloon angioplasty procedure gave Mary temporary relief, but within twelve weeks after she returned home, the vessel was closing again, and the chest pain returned. Another angioplasty was done, this time with a stint. Now, Mary was advised that she would almost certainly need bypass surgery.

That's when she came to me. She had already read my book, because with a strong family history of heart disease she wanted to learn more about protecting her family from a similar fate. Now that she was the victim herself, she had expected her cardiologist to offer serious dietary counseling. The doctor's dietitian, however, only suggested that she eat less red meat, more poultry and fish. She was given the USDA's food pyramid, which was designed, they said, to keep her calories from fat around 30 percent.

Mary wanted a more vigorous plan to reduce her dietary fat. Furthermore, she had correctly assumed that her cholesterol level of 210 mg/dl was too high, even though the cardiologist and dietitian seemed comfortable with it. Both seemed virtually certain that she would need a bypass, because the chest pain was beginning to reappear during routine physical activity.

Mary, always slender, hadn't worried about her own heart until that fateful day on the transcontinental flight. Until then, her concern was more for her family. She had eaten a typical American diet since childhood, and for the last twenty years most of her meals had been purchased in airports and hotels. Now, her own life was at stake, and she wondered why she wasn't given a more aggressive dietary approach. She had remembered reading in my book that at least six clinical studies had shown a progression of coronary lesions among victims of heart disease who consumed 30 percent of their calories as fat.

We talked at length about the proven regression of coronary lesions reported by Dr. Dean Ornish among his patients on a strict diet of vegetables, fruits, grains and legumes. I wasn't sure that Mary would comply with this, since she was a gourmet cook at home, and on the road had always eaten a relatively high-fat diet. But Mary proved me wrong. Highly motivated, and desiring not to "have my chest opened," she passionately took on my recommended *Four Stages to an Ideal Diet.* Though it was designed for gradually reducing dietary fat and animal protein over a three to four month period, she reached Stage Four within a week. Mary was now on a plant-based diet and walked briskly for thirty minutes daily. "Can I do more?" she asked.

My colleague, Dr. Caldwell Esselstyn of the Cleveland Clinic, had for several years kept me posted on a group of his patients with severe coronary artery disease, treated not only with an all plant-based diet, but also with a cholesterol-lowering drug. On this regime, his patients had much more regression of their coronary artery lesions than that reported in the literature from a plant-based diet alone. The key to this surprising degree of regression seemed to be the reduction of cholesterol levels to 150 mg/dl or below.

Mary had nothing to lose and a great deal to gain; so we convinced her cardiologist to add Lovastatin, a cholesterol-lowering drug which reduces the production of cholesterol in the liver, to her new program of diet and exercise. "It's my life," Mary said. "I can handle the dietary changes, but if the Lovastatin will add to my chance of success, I want to do it."

We were all delighted when, after four weeks, Mary's cholesterol level was 130. She felt wonderful and the chest pains did not return.

The cavalier attitude of the cardiologists and cardiac surgeons about alternative non-surgical approaches to her disease continues to dismay her. Now a strong advocate for plant-based diets for both children and adults, she has adapted many of the recipes from books by

Ornish, Pritikin, Barnard, McDougall and Attwood to her own dishes.

"I'm lucky," she said to me several months later. "Women my age don't realize that we account for half of the 500,000 coronary disease deaths every year." She's right. Heart disease is the leading cause of disability and death among women Mary's age, while breast cancer, which gets all the media attention, is a distant second.

ASK DR. ATTWOOD

Q: In planning vegan meals from the multitude of recipe books that I have seen or magazines that I have read, I still have no information how to properly plan with nutrition in mind. As an example: What should be the percentage of carbohydrates, starches, protein for a meal?

A: The wonderful thing about a plant-based (or vegan) diet is that counting calories, grams of fat, grams of carbohydrate, grams of protein, looking up vitamin and mineral content is all unnecessary. The plant-based food—a reasonable variety of fruits, vegetables, whole grains and legumes— does it all for you naturally. All the ingredients are in the right range for good health. The old adage of careful food combining for proper protein amount and quality has been considered a myth for about twenty years now.

NINE

OBESITY TRENDS AND GENES

The obesity trend among Baby Boomers skyrocketed during the closing years of the twentieth century. In order to understand this trend it is necessary to first understand that adults do not suddenly become obese. Like most other health risks, obesity usually has its beginnings during childhood, when lifelong eating patterns and physical activity habits are established. Parents' lifestyles strongly influence those of their children, who later as adults continue this vicious cycle.

Benji had been coming to our clinic for almost three months, always with his aunt, because his mother and father both worked during my office hours. At age ten, Benji tipped the scales at 140 pounds, approximately double his ideal weight. We learned early in our sessions that he spent three hours watching TV each day after school, before his parents got home. His first task, after turning on the TV, was finding a snack—usually there were cookies, candy or leftover desserts in the house. After dinner, which was often brought home by his parents from a fast-food restaurant, Benji did his homework and played video games before bedtime.

Like his parents, Benji's breakfast usually consisted of sweet rolls or a donut, since everyone was in a hurry to leave the house and get to work and school. By lunchtime Benji was famished when he got to the school cafeteria. He grabbed french fries and either a hamburger or hot dog, a glass of milk, and whatever dessert he could find. He often ate his friends' desserts. After school this cycle was repeated. Benji's daily diet was usually rounded out by several high-fat snacks between meals.

Unusual? No, actually Benji's lifestyle is typical of children his age in America and many other Western nations. A recent report by the Center for Disease Control and Prevention showed, not unexpectedly, that the incidence of severe obesity among children of Benji's age has doubled since 1965. The reason? Inactivity and a diet too high in fat and calories.

Obesity is usually a family pattern. Since children tend to adopt the eating and activity habits of their parents, if one parent is overweight, the chances of a child having a weight problem is 40 percent. If both parents are overweight, the child's chances of gaining excessive weight increases to 80 percent.

When we finally met Benji's parents, both, as we had predicted, were extremely heavy. Their attitude about his weight was best expressed by his mother: "We're not really worried," she said, "he'll probably slim down as he gets older. His cousins did."

Unfortunately, the odds are overwhelming that Benji will, without dietary and exercise intervention, become an overweight adult. Furthermore, slimming down later may not totally prevent some of the diseases associated with obesity—chiefly heart disease, stroke and cancer. A startling study at Tufts University in 1993 showed that an overweight adolescent will have an increased risk of dying prematurely of one of these major diseases before age seventy, as compared to his peers of normal weight. And surprisingly, the study showed that this increased risk is permanent—it's not corrected if the weight is later lost during the teens or adulthood.

Why should this be the case? One likely reason: excess numbers of fat cells are created during infancy and again during the years around adolescence. These are permanent throughout adulthood, always ready to serve for body-fat storage. This is the likely reason some of us are burdened with "creeping weight gains" as we age. And body-fat percentage may have a tendency to remain high, even after weight returns to normal. So, although other health risk-factors, such as high blood pressure and elevated cholesterol levels may be silent and unrecognized, obesity is obvious—the earliest visible sign of ills to come.

Lost: 22,000 Seats In Yankee Stadium!

One of the most graphic examples of increasing obesity in the U.S. is the disappearing seats of a famous baseball park. Yankee Stadium was built during the 1920s. It had about 82,000 seats. After remodeling during the 1970s the seating was only 59,000. During that fifty-year period, between Babe Ruth and such baseball greats as Thurman Munson, Ron Guidry and Reggie

Jackson, the average American "bottom" had widened from fourteen inches to nineteen inches. Today, patrons at the Mickey Mantle Restaurant in New York, where a few of the original seats were installed, have found them to be a tight fit.

It's Not The Genes

In 1996 the Center for Disease Control and Prevention reported that obesity is far more common today than it was just thirty years ago. For the first time in history, according to Federal Body Mass Index (BMI) standards, there are more overweight people in the United States than people of normal weight. The aging Baby Boomers have become known as the generation of obesity. Let's take another look at their lifestyle.

Aren't we eating less fat? And what about all those selections of fat-free snacks and other foods flying off the supermarket shelves? We forget that all those fat-free foods are not necessarily low in calories. One of my patients admitted to consuming 1,000 calories from a package of fat-free fig cookies before she reached the checkout counter of her supermarket.

Portion and serving sizes are getting larger also, not just in the supermarket, but in fast food restaurants. Serving sizes in France, for example, are usually much smaller than in this country. Most Europeans, in fact, are astonished by the size of our hamburgers, pizzas, servings of popcorn and soft drinks. Predictably, the rate of obesity among the French and Europeans in general is much less than in this country, even though they consume as much or more fat than Americans.

So, why do we find ourselves getting fatter year after year? The common answer given by most people, as well as most health care professionals is disturbing. Because if they're right, nothing can be done about this terrible health risk, which according to former Surgeon General C. Everett Koop, is second only to smoking as a cause of premature death.

"It's the genes," people say. "Our family is just that way." But think about it. During the past thirty years the genetic pattern of U.S. citizens couldn't have changed—this takes thousands of years. Yet obesity has increased by over 30 percent during a scant three decades.

A fifty-billion-dollar diet industry in the United States unwisely bases its programs primarily on caloric restriction; and its failure rate is high. We learned from the China Health Study that people living in rural Chinese ingest 30 percent more calories than we do, yet obesity is rare among them. More physical activity and a plant-based diet with little fat and animal protein seem to be the answer to this paradox. These two factors apparently work together to increase the "resting metabolism." At total rest, or even sleep, a person with a higher metabolic resting-rate burns more calories per hour than a person with a lower rate. The human body is genetically programmed to behave this way.

Ironically, our overeating and inadequate exercise habits extend even to family pets. Veterinarian Joseph Killian, now retired in Southern California, observed during his many years of practice that overweight families usually owned overweight pets.

Obesity is serious. Let's face it; it's due to lifestyle habits—excessive calories and inactivity—but *not* our genes. The father is fat, the mother is fat, the child is fat, and the family dog is fat.

ASK DR. ATTWOOD

Q : My daughter, husband and grandparents are all overweight. Several members of the family developed diabetes during their middle years. I'm the only slender person in our family. How much do you think their genes play in this tendency to gain weight and get diabetes? What can I expect for my grandchildren?

A : I'm inclined to believe that obesity is usually determined for the most part by lifestyle, and to a far lesser extent by genetic factors. During the past decade the incidence of obesity has doubled, whereas the human genetic pattern hasn't changed for over 50,000 years.

Even when there may be a slight genetic tendency to gain weight, this is far outweighed by eating and exercise patterns. Adult onset diabetes is another example. We know that there is a genetic tendency to develop this disease among certain individuals who gain excessive weight. A proper plant-based diet and exercise program effectively prevents obesity, and the gene may never express itself. In other words, lifestyle habits almost always outperform genes.

Q: I'm a divorced single mom and raise my six-year-old daughter vegan during the week. But on the weekend my husband is feeding her hamburgers and fish sticks. She comes home with an upset stomach every Sunday evening. She's also started putting on some weight. Is there anything I can do about this?

A: In my book, *Dr. Attwood's Low-Fat Prescription for Kids* (Penguin,1995), Chapter 21—which was written by Victoria Moran—gives good advice on this issue. Victoria suggests first trying to get your ex-spouse on your side, by convincing him of the health risk of high-fat, animal-based foods. He needs to understand why a plant-based diet is best for your daughter's future health. Give him a copy of the book. Hopefully, he'll be converted by the time he finishes the introduction.

"In the meanwhile, make whatever subtle but important changes you can," Victoria says, "and keep the overall picture in mind. Your children are what they eat, but they're a lot more than that as well. Their health also depends on exercise, adequate rest and sleep, fresh air, and more subtle elements such as feeling loved and worthy."

Concerning parents living together with this discord, she adds, "I am convinced that having a stable family life without parental discord over a daily issue like 'what's for dinner?' is more significant than whether a child's diet contains 15 per-

cent of calories from fat or 25 during the transi-
tional stages."

A VEGETARIAN DOCTOR SPEAKS OUT

TEN

WINE WITH DINNER?

R elax. If you enjoy a glass or two of wine with dinner I'm not going to spoil your life. Moderate consumption of alcohol, whether wine, beer or liqueur has consistently been related to a decreased risk of heart disease in clinical studies, almost without exception. This has been attributed to various effects of alcohol, including its antioxidant properties (the fact that it tends to raise the protective HDL cholesterol levels), as well as its relationship to relaxation and social connections. Combined, I am sure these are significant, but the real relationship between alcohol consumption and a lower risk of heart disease is much simpler and provable: the anticoagulant effect.

Alcohol slightly delays or inhibits the coagulation of blood. Ninety-five percent of heart attacks are brought on by a blood clot that finishes the total occlusion of an already narrowed coronary artery. This bleeding usually comes from a rupture of the cholesterol plaque in the vessel, and anything that inhibits this clot formation may actually prevent the total occlusion of the vessel.

There are several ways, other than alcohol, to inhibit clotting. Drugs, known as anticoagulants, are rarely used in healthy individuals. Aspirin's anticoagulative effect has made it a favorite among physicians and cardiologists for their patients. Vitamin E seems to have such an effect as does the Omega 3 of fish oil. Another commonly overlooked and natural way to create an anticoagulant effect is by simple aerobic exercise.

Alcohol, in moderation, with the vitamin E obtained naturally in foods, such as wheat germ, corn, asparagus, spinach, broccoli, kale, Brussel sprouts, cucumber and whole-grain cereals, along with aerobic exercise, would seem to me to be complimentary and healthy without the use of aspirin or fish oils. The key here is alcohol in moderation, considered by most authorities as two drinks daily or less.

A few caveats: I would never recommend alcoholic beverages to anyone who does not already consume them regularly, or suggest an increase in consumption to anyone who may only occasionally imbibe. The risk of alcoholism and abuse of this substance is real, and would far outweigh any protection that may be received against heart disease. I would caution anyone with chronic liver disease against consuming any alcoholic beverages.

So relax. Your one or two glasses of wine with dinner are perfectly compatible with a vegetarian lifestyle.

ASK DR. ATTWOOD

Q: For a number of years now I have noticed a distinct pain in my lower back in the kidney area following consumption the previous day of wine or alcohol, which could be described in the medium-to-heavy consumption range. The only way to get relief from this pain is to abstain from alcohol and consume large quantities of cranberry juice.

I recently consulted a homeopathic physician who diagnosed inflammation of the kidney caused by an allergy to citric acid and tartaricum acidum, which he said was found in white wines. What do you think?

A: I would strongly advise that you limit your alcohol consumption. Anything exceeding one drink a day for women and two for men has regularly caused a direct irritant effect upon the kidneys and especially, the bladder. Drink lots of water. I do not relate this to an allergy to citric acid, just an irritant effect of the alcohol.

ELEVEN

CONTROLLING FOOD ALLERGIES

A Pound of Prevention

I was a severe asthmatic throughout my childhood, and often missed several days of school each month. On many occasions this was complicated by pneumonia or bronchitis, when I would be hospitalized and placed in an oxygen tent. My parents felt helpless, and I'm sure our doctor shared their concern. The only known treatment was an injection (sometimes several) of adrenaline, when the gasping and wheezing got severe, and antibiotics, usually penicillin, for secondary infections. We were usually offered the encouraging words, "At least it won't kill you."

In retrospect, I now understand that this was the doctor's attempt to compensate for his inability to deal with this miserable disease. I'm certain that it never occurred to him, or to my parents, that my asthma may have been caused by something that I was eating; or that it may have been preventable.

Even now, I can still remember the sensation of being unable to get enough air into and out of my lungs, though I haven't had asthma since leaving home for college at age seventeen. Many years later, during my pediatric specialty training, I made the connection: Milk and dairy products, which I never really liked, had been discontinued when I left home for college. During the following years, as a practicing pediatrician, I would see this relationship of asthma, and several other allergic disorders, to dairy products time and time again.

After seeing two generations of my patients struggle with this malady, I've come to the conclusion—which is now shared by many allergists—that six out of ten children are allergic to milk protein. Not all are asthmatics; many have recurrent middle-ear infections, allergic rhinitis and, especially in infants, chronic skin rashes such as eczema. Older children and adults often manifest their food-related allergies as chronic bronchitis and sinusitis. But asthma itself may persist for a lifetime.

Milk and dairy products aren't the only foods capable of causing severe allergies in children and adults. Others are eggs, seafood, soybeans, peanuts, corn, tomatoes and wheat, to name a few. Allergic disorders are caused by proteins known as allergens, so they're commonly associated with foods of high protein content, especially of animal origin. Remembering my experience as a child, I've always discontinued dairy products as a first step for my severely allergic patients, before going on to a full allergic work-up. This simple approach often surprises the whole family, who have been used to sleepless nights and the constant and disappointing use of aerosol inhalations, shots and drugs.

"Why hasn't this simple approach been done before?" they ask. Good question. I've had dozens of severe asthmatics who have been treated by physicians unsuccessfully for years. Many physicians are, unfortunately, trained only to treat illnesses; they're not as inclined to approach allergies as a preventable disorder.

More protein may mean more allergies, as the following chart indicates:

Protein in Grams per Serving

Corn, (3 1/2 oz)..3
Milk, skim (8 oz)..8
Eggs (2)..12
Soybeans (1/2 cup cooked)....................17
Brazil nuts (3 1/2 oz).............................14
Shrimp (3 1/2 oz)..................................21
Peanuts (3 1/2 oz)................................26
Pork (3 1/2 oz)......................................30

The attitude that ignores or overlooks the relationship between diet and allergies may necessarily change in the near future because the number of asthma deaths has risen sharply during the last decade, both in this country and in Europe. The increasing use of repeated doses, sometimes daily, of such drugs as Albuterol, a bronchial dilator, has corresponded to this increase in fatalities, especially in the inner cities of the U.S. Again, this is a failure of using a treatment approach rather than using prevention.

Since asthma is an allergic disease in most cases, and

involves a secondary inflammatory change in the bronchioles, the use of inhaled corticosteroids is becoming a standard medical procedure for severe asthmatics as a prevention of serious attacks of wheezing. This has been more effective than waiting for the shortness of breath to begin, but obviously does nothing to eliminate the underlying cause.

Food is not the only allergen-containing material that precipitates asthma and the other allergic diseases. Inhalants, such as house dust mites, molds, the excretions of cockroaches, and pollens often play an important role. Many individuals are allergic to several foods as well as several inhalants. Unlike food, many of these inhalants cannot easily be avoided, so there may be a need for weekly desensitizing injections of an extract which contains gradually increasing doses of these offending substances. Food allergies are simpler to prevent; after they're identified, they're just avoided. Sounds simple? It was, until March of 1996, when stories about genetically-engineered foods began appearing on the front pages of newspapers throughout the country.

Genetic engineering of foods, another trick against Mother Nature, is almost certain to bring with it mass confusion about food allergies. The first attempts to introduce the genes of Brazil nuts—with its over 1000 proteins—into soybeans, were successful in creating a more protein-dense soybean. But the thousands of people who were allergic to Brazil nuts would, according to early clinical testing, be allergic to this new variety of "super soybean." A likely moratorium may halt this new product until the allergy consequences are fully known. But we can be assured that this is only the beginning;

food manufacturers are planning to introduce these new superfoods by the hundreds, each containing the genes of many other plant species. Preventing food allergies will then be possible only when consumers make their choices from labeled "organically-grown" foods.

The key to food-allergy management still remains the same. We must follow nature's rules and prevent them, rather than treat them. Why go on living with these disorders, allowing them to reappear regularly, and then try to treat them, always with questionable results? It's certainly a bit hasty to immediately go through a comprehensive allergic work-up involving skin testing. Save this for later. First, pick the top food allergens—dairy products, eggs, meat, seafood, soybeans, corn, and wheat—and remove them from the diet, one at a time, for four to six weeks, beginning first with dairy products. This can be done with the help of a food diary—a daily log of food eaten and the frequency of symptoms.

Now, back to that villain that causes the majority of allergic disorders: milk and other dairy products. Here again, always take the simplest step first. It's usually unnecessary to avoid every conceivable food that contains the slightest amount of dairy products. Fortunately, small amounts cooked with other foods, and in commercial products, are often well tolerated. Just remove the obvious sources of milk, cheese and yogurt from the diet. If you are rewarded with noticeable improvement, then you can refine the procedure by carefully reading labels. Talk with your pediatrician or family physician. Tell him you're ready for a pound of prevention.

ASK DR. ATTWOOD

Q: I have an eighteen-month-old and a four-month-old. Both drank breast-milk for three weeks, then were switched to Similac® with iron. My commitment to the Air Force as a pilot prevented me from any type of pumping to insure they both had breast-milk after I returned to work.

At age one, my older child started drinking whole milk. I have been a vegetarian for fifteen years, always striving to remain vegan. However, I was concerned about that one-to-two-year-old period. If I could breast-feed I would, but is soy milk really okay for my toddler after that first year? I have probably fallen victim to my Midwestern dairy/meat upbringing.

A: When possible, breast-feed for at least one year. Then forget the bottle or formulas and go on to soft (blended) table food. Milk (whole, soy, etc) is not needed. Whenever you cannot breast-feed, soy is the only sensible alternative, never a cow's milk formula. I suggest soy reluctantly, because infants seem to be getting sensitized (allergic) to soy and unable to tolerate it later in life.

The same scenario is possible (directly to soft

foods) if parents could breast-feed as long as six months.

❧❧❧

Q: Eight years ago, at age thirty-eight, I had several severe attacks of hives that sent me to the emergency room. At the time I ate red meat infrequently and was able to find a pattern in these occurrences. I have stopped eating all beef and pork and have had no problems.

What am I allergic to? Is it the meat itself, an antibiotic, or other drug given to the livestock, or something else? Would it be safe to have organic meat?

A: Any high protein food, whether animal or plant, can cause severe allergic reactions. Of course, some other substance given to the cattle could be responsible, but I wouldn't risk it. Actually, your diet would be much healthier without these high-fat, high-animal protein sources, regardless of the allergic reactions.

TWELVE

IS IT REALLY ATTENTION DEFICIT DISORDER?

Or Does Food Change Behavior?

Brian, age six, didn't show one moment of shyness when he and his mother entered my examining room. In fact, after five minutes he had already turned on the water at the lavatory, inspected the pictures on the wall (knocking several off their hooks), and examined the entire contents of the wastebasket in the corner. His mother handed me a note from his first grade teacher. Brian, it said, distracted the whole class, couldn't stay in his seat, and behaved in a manner much like I was witnessing at that moment.

Many parents, like Brian's, have been contacted by school authorities about learning difficulties their children have encountered in the classroom, or of behavior problems at school. Parents wonder, "Is it serious or is it just a phase?"

You may know such families, and you may want to help. Perhaps you remember reading about a condition known as Attention Deficit Disorder (ADD), which has appeared frequently in the news media in recent years.

It's a poorly understood affliction characterized by an abnormally short attention span and often, but not always, hyperactivity, when it's then called Attention Deficit Hyperactivity Disorder (ADHD). I now see more of these children in my office each day than I saw in a whole month fifteen years ago. Fortunately, ADD and ADHD can be successfully managed in most cases, but first a definite diagnosis must be made.

Where does a parent begin? What about special testing and treatment? Pediatrician Mike Melancon of Lafayette, Louisiana, who specializes in the diagnosis and treatment of ADD, asked parents at a recent seminar, "Does everyone have ADD? Does anyone have it?" He admits that he still doesn't know for sure. In my experience, it's a real entity, classically starting very early in childhood, during infancy, and often continuing throughout the teens and even into adulthood. Parents of these children generally recall a very active infant and preschooler. The Parent-Teacher Questionnaire below is a sensible first step in diagnosing this disorder.

My brief test can be carried out by a parent at home, and then by a teacher who has observed the child regularly in a classroom. This adaptation of material first published by Dr. Keith Conners is a modification of a more comprehensive psychological test, with questions pertaining to ADD and ADHD grouped and easily arranged for a parent and a teacher to score. The following test is only a guideline, of course; the child's doctor will have to make the final diagnosis.

DIRECTIONS:
Use two copies of the test below—one for the evalu-

ating parent, one for the child's teacher. The parent and teacher should not see the other's scores before making an evaluation. Based on his or her assessment of the child's behavior, each evaluator assigns a numerical score to each of the ten qualities listed.

Scores: 0 = not at all, 1 = just a little, 2 = pretty much, and 3 = very much.

PARENT'S EVALUATION

1.Excitable, impulsive ( )

2.Difficulty in learning ( )

3.Restless, squirmy ( )

4.Restless, on the go ( )

5.Doesn't finish things ( )

6.Childish, immature ( )

7.Short attention span ( )

8.Easily frustrated ( )

9.Quick mood changes ( )

10.Denies mistakes ( )

Total ( )

TEACHER'S EVALUATION

1.Excitable, impulsive ( )

2.Difficulty in learning ( )

3.Restless, squirmy ( )

4.Restless, on the go ( )

5.Doesn't finish things ( )

6.Childish, immature ( )

7.Short attention span ( )

8.Easily frustrated ( )

9.Disturbs other children ( )

10.Demands quick attention ( )

Total ( )

Combined total ( )

SCORING: Add up the total score of the parent's questionnaire.

Add up the total score of the teacher's questionnaire.

Now add the two scores together for a Combined total. If the combined total is 36 or more, there is a high probability that the child has attention deficit disorder and could benefit from treatment.

Scores of 15 by the parent alone or 15 by the teacher alone should be considered a possibility. Take these scores to your doctor for his or her opinion.

☙❧

What causes this perplexing condition, and why are we seeing so much more of it than ever before? One of the major controversies concerning ADD today is whether or not food additives, food colorings, preservatives, sugar (sucrose), or aspartame either cause it or make is more pronounced. A double-blind controlled study conducted by the Department of Pediatrics at Vanderbilt University, and reported in the *New England Journal of Medicine* (Feb. 1994), found no evidence that either sugar or aspartame affected children's behavior or cognitive function, even though the study group had been described by the parents as being sensitive to sugar.

Another 1994 study at the University of Melbourne, Australia, reported in the *Royal Journal of Pediatrics*, found a strong association between hyperactivity and a synthetic food coloring (tartrazine). This double-blind study also reported increasing hyperactivity throughout six increasing dose levels of the dye. Still, other clinical studies have shown no relationship between ADD and sugar, food colorings, or any other food additive.

Chronic lead poisoning and the fetal alcohol syndrome have also been suggested as possible causes of this disorder. However, in the great majority of my cases, this etiology has been ruled out. Whatever the cause, in my experience, the condition is more or less permanent, extending well into adulthood.

An interesting improvement of irritability and other negative mood states, including tobacco withdrawal and premenstrual syndrome, by a diet high in complex carbohydrates has been reported consistently in the medical literature. But the possibility that inattention and hyperactivity in either children or adults may be caused or worsened by a high animal protein intake—a characteristic of the typical American diet—has not been adequately studied.

ADD, carefully diagnosed by professionals, seems to have the unique characteristic of sudden and dramatic improvement when treated by certain stimulant drugs, such as Ritalin, Dexadrine, Adderol or Clyert. If a medical professional wishes to treat this condition with any of these medications, the questionnaire above may be used to follow the progress of treatment, and for making adjustments in dosage. Sometimes the effect of Ritalin is incredible. I've very often seen children go from failing grades to the Dean's List within a month. Ongoing counseling by a therapist familiar with the disorder seems to enhance any effects from medication.

And finally, I've concluded during recent years that my patients who are on a plant-based diet for high cholesterol levels or obesity rarely have severe ADD. Those who do seem to respond more easily to treatment, whether it be Ritalin or counseling or both. The dietary approach, in my opinion, should precede the others. Once again, my *Four Stages to an Ideal Diet* (see page107) is a sensible first step.

ASK DR. ATTWOOD

Q: My wife has an anxiety disorder. Any help you could offer would be greatly appreciated.

A: Drugs are rarely the final answer to anxiety states. A high complex-carbohydrate diet has always been associated with mellow behavior, pacifism, etc. I've found it helpful for children who have Attention Deficit Disorder and Hyperactivity.

I would also encourage prolonged aerobic activity. It can be very moderate, but when prolonged (forty-five minutes or so), there is a definite anti-anxiety effect.

A VEGETARIAN DOCTOR SPEAKS OUT

THIRTEEN

VITAMIN B-12

Should You Worry?

Isabella, my granddaughter, is now three years old. She has never tasted meat or milk. She was breastfed for the first year and then went directly to a variety of vegetables, fruits and grains. Nevertheless, her physical growth and development, according to the Denver Developmental Scale, is well above average. She has the smoothest skin I've ever seen—none of the rough areas of eczema usually seen in infants. Isabella also doesn't have ear infections, wheezing or other respiratory illness seen so often in milk drinkers. "Where does she get vitamin B-12?" her regular pediatrician asks. He pointed out—correctly at the time—that B-12 was only found in animal products. The answer, for now, is that she gets it from the breast milk she had during her first year of life. Her mother recently asked me whether or not a supplement will be necessary as she gets older. So let's look at some older vegetarians to see how they deal with the B-12 dilemma.

Ocean Robbins, of Santa Cruz, California, the twenty-five-year-old son of EarthSave founder John Robbins, has never eaten meat, and for the past ten years he has consumed no animal products whatsoever. Yet, his physical growth has always been above average and he's rarely been sick. Ocean excelled in both sports and academics throughout his childhood, setting elementary school records for pull-ups, push-ups and the 10 km run for ten-year-olds. He and his father, another famed vegetarian, together recently ran a full marathon. Both take B-12 supplements daily, which, Ocean reminds me, don't come from animal sources.

Dick Gregory, the great stand-up comic and civil rights leader, has been a vegetarian since 1964. His physical endurance, which has been proven by several ultra-long distance walks, has not diminished during the past three decades. At age sixty-four, Dick Gregory remains extremely physically active and hasn't been ill in many years. When I asked if he took supplements containing B-12, he said, "Oh yes, quite a few."

Isabella's Recommended Daily Allowance (RDA) for this vitamin, known to be necessary for cell division and blood formation, is estimated by the National Research Council to be 1 microgram (0.001 mg). The RDA for Ocean and Dick should be about 2 micrograms (0.002 mg). However, millions of people worldwide have no known source for this amount of B-12, yet they remain perfectly healthy. So where is it coming from? Are there any plant sources?

Readers of Frances Moore Lappé's *Diet for a Small Planet* may remember reading in its first edition (1971) that certain fermented soy products, such as tempeh and miso, and seaweed contained vitamin B-12. These sources have recently been shown to contain only the inactive analogue of the vitamin, not metabolized by humans. Ironically, they may actually interfere with the metabolism of active B-12.

The American Academy of Pediatrics' Committee on Nutrition states that deficiencies of vitamin B-12 (known chemically as cobalomin), which are extremely serious, and may ultimately lead to irreversible nerve damage, are rarely found among vegetarian children or adults throughout the world. The rural Chinese for example, some of whom consume only vegetables, fruits and grains (persons eating no animal products whatsoever are known as *vegans*) show no symptoms attributable to deficiencies of this vitamin. So the risk is not great.

Personally, during forty years of pediatric practice, I've never encountered a single case of B-12 deficiency. Yet, most of my colleagues who advocate a plant-based diet are somewhat cautious and recommend some source of B-12. Dr. Dean Ornish suggests an occasional cup of skim milk. Dr. Neal Barnard recommends taking a multi-vitamin or B-12 fortified foods.

The most likely explanation for this extreme rarity of B-12 deficiencies among vegans is a process I will call "self-synthesis." Since bacteria from the soil on plants consumed by animals produce B-12 within their gastrointestinal tracts, it's reasonable to assume that the same may happen when individuals eat natural foods. This is more likely if the plants are not carefully cleaned, not washed, or overcooked.

The Vegetarian Resource Group states—tongue-in-cheek, I suspect—that some vegans may get B-12 from "just not washing their hands," but they are quick to point out that this isn't a reliable source. Also, it's been suggested that B-12, like iron, may be absorbed more efficiently by vegans than by people consuming animal products.

Furthermore, a little of this vitamin goes a long, long way. The body can store it for at least five years, and probably much longer. There are virtually always adequate amounts for anyone who even occasionally consumes B-12 sources. In fact, according to B-12 researcher Victor Herbert, M.D., at New York's Mount Sinai Medical Center, there's evidence that vegans who previously ate animal-based food may have vitamin B-12 stores that will not be depleted for up to twenty years.

Reports occasionally still appear, most recently from Europe, that plants may contain B-12, especially if fertilized organically with cow dung, commonly referred to in this country as manure. These studies aren't convincing, and I will reserve judgement about active B-12 in plant tissue until I see more evidence.

In summary, it seems that vegetarians who consume enough calories face very little chance of developing a B-12 deficiency. But let's face it, parents would like total assurance that they and their children will not be at risk. For them, I would suggest a multivitamin containing B-12 or a fortified breakfast cereal, soy milk, or meat substitute. Some forms of nutritional yeast contain adequate amounts of B-12. These non-animal sources are fine; just read the labels.

Then you can go ahead and wash your hands.

ASK DR. ATTWOOD

Q: I was diagnosed with B–12 deficiency several years ago. After testing, my physician told me that I am not capable of absorbing B–12 and that I will need injections for the rest of my life. My questions is: Is there something I can do to improve my B–12 absorption? Should I take supplements or eat a lot of foods high in B–12 along with the shots? Should I be tested periodically to see if the situation was temporary and has changed?

I am a lacto-vegetarian (presently eating 2/3 cup of nonfat cottage cheese daily, which I intend to give up when I can find a recipe for a "mock version").

A: Your diet seems adequate. I wouldn't necessarily change it. Your B–12 absorption problem may be permanent and require the injections. The condition you may have is pernicious anemia, which is the absence of "Castle's intrinsic factor," which is necessary for the absorption of B–12. It would have been almost impossible on your present diet to become deficient in this vitamin due to lack of it. In fact, it would take fifteen to twenty years to become deficient in B–12 if all sources of animal products were totally absent in the food you eat.

FOURTEEN

A NEW LOOK AT THE SOYBEAN

Still Great—But Not A Panacea

The soybean, judging from comments by my colleagues, patients and readers, seems to have attained the status of a matinee idol—almost always the hero. Occasionally, and not unexpectedly due to its constant aura of mystique, it has been cast in the role of a villain. But stardom didn't come overnight for this mainstay of the Asian diet, which was considered by the ancient Chinese to be one of the five sacred grains, along with rice, wheat, barley and millet. Soybeans date back to 2838 B.C.E. in China, the sixth century in Japan, and the seventeenth century in Europe.

Despite the soybean's bland flavor, the United States became interested in the 1920s, when its full nutrient value and inexpensive production were finally appreciated. Now our country grows one third of the total world supply, mostly for livestock feed and non-food commercial products. Surprisingly, only 2 percent is destined for human consumption, in the form of soybean oil, tempeh, miso, tofu, soy milk, soy flour, soy sauce and the dried bean. Fresh soybeans are not generally available except in Asian markets or specialty produce markets in late summer and early fall.

The soybean may have been a lifesaver for certain groups of people and at times in world history when calories were inadequate. Examples include the POWs of World War II, and more recently, the residents of Cuba during the thirty-six-year embargo. In both instances, the soybean was credited with preventing starvation and death. Its value is no less in calorie-rich societies, such as the United States and most Western countries, where soybeans, like oat bran, have been shown to reduce cholesterol levels when replacing animal proteins in the diet. This is probably due to its richness in soluble fiber and the fact that it replaces some of the saturated fat in the diet.

Because of the soybean's high protein content, many individuals have been under the impression that a proper plant-based diet *must* include soy products, in combination with other "less complete" protein sources. Unfortunately, in this respect, the famous bean has probably frightened away some individuals who would have benefited from a meatless diet. Patients in my clinic often say that the prospect of rounding out their daily menu with tempeh or tofu is not exactly appetizing.

Vegetarianism, in general, may have been somewhat tainted by this soy association for decades. As discussed in a previous essay, Frances Moore Lappé, in her 1971 groundbreaking book, *Diet for a Small Planet*, dispelled the myth that meat was needed for complete protein. Her solution of carefully combining vegetable proteins was retracted in the 1991 edition. She admitted that it "reinforced another myth," and asserted that, "If people are getting enough calories, they are virtually certain of getting enough protein." Lappé's sample plant-based menu, which exceeded the protein requirements of the National Academy of Sciences, contained no soy products. In recent years it has been found that such careful food-combining isn't necessary. Frances was right!

Her best seller—over three million sold, and still selling—also popularized the concept that fermented soy products, such as tempeh and miso, contained significant amounts of vitamin B-12. But more recent assays show that this is an inactive B-12 analogue, not utilized as the vitamin in human consumption; and according to some investigators, may block actual B-12 metabolism.

Suzanne Havala, M.S.,R.D., author of the American Dietetic Association's 1992 position paper on vegetarian diets and the new book, *Shopping For Health*, recently told me, "It isn't necessary that people who dislike miso, tofu, or tempeh have to eat them or other soy products in order to get adequate quality proteins." Havala agrees that a variety of plant matter will do as long as the individual consumes enough calories. "Soy products," she said, "on the other hand, are nutrient-dense and a very good choice." She adds that their taste has improved in recent years and she doesn't personally consider them bland.

Like any legume, the soybean is nutrient-packed, but unlike other beans, there may be a few caveats to consider before eating unlimited amounts of soy products. First, in my practice I have found that allergies to the soybean are far more common than to other legumes. Newborn infants seem to tolerate commercial soy formulas very well, but according to the American Academy of Pediatrics, this early exposure may be causing some of the soy allergies I'm now seeing in older children and adults. Pediatric allergist Brent Prather of Lafayette, Louisiana agrees. He tells me he sees far more soy allergies in children than his pediatrician father did before commercial soy formulas came into common use in the 1960s.

Second, soybeans are 60 percent oil and a significant source of fat that can add as much as 9 grams per serving (one-half cup cooked beans or a three-and-one-half ounce block of tofu)—one sixth of it's fat is saturated. When combined with other ingredients in American dishes, soy typically adds about 5 grams of fat per serving.

And finally, some recent reports suggest that precipitated soy products, such as tofu, if consumed regularly, may inhibit the absorption of such minerals as calcium, magnesium, iron and especially zinc.

The word "soybean" on a food label doesn't always mean good nutrition. Often, the opposite may be the case. Soybean oil is used in hundreds of processed foods, especially snacks, salad dressings and margarine, in a partially hydrogenated form (see the next essay) made more saturated by adding hydrogen atoms. This altered version, known as a trans-fatty acid, is everywhere—in graham crackers, Ginger Snaps®, even SnackWells®. Like natural saturated fat, soybean oil appears to raise cholesterol levels, but also lowers HDL. Here, one should watch the ingredient portion of food labels—hydrogenated oils are not identified alongside total and saturated fat.

In summary, even though the soybean is an excellent source of protein and fiber—and a good choice—it's no panacea, and isn't mandatory for a well-balanced, plant-based diet. Complete, high-quality vegetable protein is assured by a variety of vegetables eaten within one day—not necessarily in one meal—assuming adequate calories are consumed.

Keeping in mind its fat content, proneness to creating allergies and possible interference with mineral absorption, let's say that a moderate consumption of soy products, along with a variety of vegetables and other legumes, would be prudent for both children and adults.

ASK DR. ATTWOOD

Q: My kids hate soy milk and ask me for regular milk. Any suggestions?

A: Rice milk is an excellent alternative. Milk can also be made from nuts, such as almonds. This is even more important now that we are seeing lots of soy allergies. Rice milk is available in most supermarkets and health-food stores. I helped produce a Telly–Award–winning video called *MOOOOOve Over Milk*, which shows how to make almond milk at home with a blender. (Inquiries: 800-453-8732)

🐄🐄🐄

Q: I am a vegetarian who is allergic to beans, especially soy. I have eczema and respiratory reactions to beans and would appreciate any suggestions on how to eliminate this problem.

A: Allergies to beans, especially soy products, are increasingly common. Their high-protein content can be allergenic. It is not necessary to eat beans or soy products on a vegetarian diet. Any reasonable variety of fruits, vegetables, and grains will provide you with adequate nutrition.

FIFTEEN

HYDROGENATED OILS: A VEGETARIAN'S PITFALL

We call them "trans-fatty acids" and they're everywhere. Margarine, crackers, cookies, cakes, doughnuts, frostings, peanut butter and practically all packaged low-fat snacks contain this unnatural food product. For over forty years the food industry has been slipping them into our processed food for firmness and increased shelf life. Many people who consider themselves healthy vegetarians are unknowingly eating trans-fats every day. We now know that they're even worse than the dreaded saturated fat of meat, butter, eggs, cheese and milk.

Trans-fatty acids are produced by adding hydrogen to a polyunsaturated oil, usually soybean oil, which makes it more saturated and firm, a process known as hydrogenation. They raise the cholesterol levels of people who consume them, just like saturated fats, but they also reduce the protective HDL cholesterol levels—this is something not even saturated fats do. A recent Harvard School of Public Health study concluded that these "hydrogenated fats" account for a significant amount of the coronary heart disease in this country. Various estimates of the proportion of heart disease caused by these hydrogenated fats, independent of the more commonly known saturated fats, range from 5 to 10 percent. Dr. Walter Willett, of the Harvard study, in a recent statement estimated that hydrogenated fat is responsible for more than 30,000 heart disease deaths per year.

To make matters worse, the current labeling law allows food processors to include these hydrogenated (trans-) fats without you and I knowing how much they're adding, because hydrogenated oils are not included in the saturated fat totals on the label. The only way you will know they're there is by reading the fine print in the ingredients part of the label and looking for the words "partially hydrogenated soybean oil" (or whatever other oil they may have used). But amounts of individual ingredients are not given on food labels.

So, let me say this: "Stay away from them!" Read labels carefully. Don't let this food industry trick undermine your otherwise healthy vegetarian diet.

ASK DR. ATTWOOD

Q: I'm underweight, and I've tried to gain weight by eating more carbohydrates (whole grains), but it hasn't work. Everyone is telling me to get more fat in my diet, however I feel uncomfortable doing this because of the risks of heart disease, cancer, etc. All the same, I really need to gain weight. Any help would be appreciated.

A: You can stay with plant-based foods while increasing calories (and even fat). Eat more nuts and soy products, if necessary, and you may want to consume vegetable oils in moderation. Be careful to avoid vegetable oils with saturated fat, however. Canola oil contains the least (only about 6 percent is saturated), while olive oil is 17 percent saturated fat. Coconut oil is by far the worst—95 percent saturated fat. And finally, if you are active and feeling well, your weight may be just fine as it is.

SIXTEEN

AN ICON SPEAKS OUT
A Final Gift

I was driving up the Maine coast with Judy Calmes (now my wife), then my publicity agent for speaking tours and co-author of an upcoming book. I was making my third visit to Dr. Benjamin Spock and his wife, Mary Morgan. It was October 1996 and the foliage was afire as far as the eye could see—the leaves were changing to bright yellows, oranges, and most spectacular of all, brilliant reds. These endless mountain forests were altering their colors just in time for our trip. This was to be a social visit combined with several more days of manuscript rewrites of *Dr. Spock's Baby and Child Care.*

The changing leaves could have been a metaphor, I thought, for other great changes that would take place over the next four days in parts of one of the greatest and most influential books of the century. I was a consultant to Dr. Spock for the rewriting of the nutrition sections of his all-time bestseller, the classic, *Baby and Child Care,* which has been a standard for parents for the past fifty years.

For the first time ever, the most famous pediatrician in the world would make drastic changes in his advice to parents about feeding their children. He would now rec- ommend a mostly vegetarian diet, and no dairy products at all for children over the age of two. I was chosen to help in this major revision, because Dr. Spock had been impressed by, and had written the Foreword for my book, *Dr. Attwood's Low-Fat Prescription For Kids* (Penguin,1995).

Dr. Spock was a vegetarian until age twelve. This led to healthy growth—six feet, four inches—and great phys- ical strength. Furthermore, he was a gold medallist at the 1924 Olympics—an event which was popularized in the movie, "Chariots of Fire." Throughout most of his long and spectacular career in medicine, politics and human rights, however, he consumed a typical high-fat American diet. But this would change drastically after a mild stroke at age eighty-eight. He then resumed his vegetarian diet, and by age ninety-four he was physically active—travel- ing, writing and speaking with a vigor and enthusiasm he had not experienced in many years.

Parents will now read in the new edition of *Baby and Child Care* that Dr. Spock was convinced that children should eat a plant-based diet—mostly vegetables, fruits, whole grains and legumes, with very little or no meat and no dairy products—to avoid the leading causes of pre- mature death later as adults: namely, heart disease, stroke, cancer and diabetes. Working with this great man, this great icon, to make those changes, was an inestimable honor for me.

You may ask how this plant-based diet can be imple- mented when most children, and most families, have already developed a strong taste for their meat, milk and cheese.

According to Dr. Spock, the answer is found in my *Four Stages to an Ideal Diet,* adapted from my first book and outlined in the chart below.

Dr. Attwood's Four Stages To An Ideal Diet

Stage 1

- Limit meat, including poultry and fish, to 3 oz. per day.

- Low-fat (1%) milk and low-fat dairy products if desired.

- No foods fried in oil.

- One dessert and one snack daily.

- Unlimited vegetables, fruits, grains and legumes.

Stage 2

- Limit trimmed meat, including skinless poultry and fish, to 3 oz. no more than three times a week.

- Skim milk and nonfat dairy foods, if desired.

- No foods fried in oil.

- One low-fat dessert and one low-fat snack daily.

- Unlimited vegetables, fruits, grains and legumes.

Stage 3

- Trimmed meat, including skinless poultry and fish, no more than 3 oz. once a week, or used sparingly as a condiment to vegetable dishes.

- Non-soy fat-free meat substitutes.

- Skim milk and non-fat dairy foods, if desired.

- No foods fried in oil.

- One fat-free dessert and one fat-free snack daily.

- Unlimited vegetables, fruits, grains, and legumes.

Stage 4

- No meat, poultry or fish.

- Unlimited vegetables, fruits, grains, and legumes.

- Non-soy fat-free meat substitutes.

- One fat-free dessert and one fat-free snack daily.

- Vitamin B–12 sources or supplements.

Adapted from: *Dr. Attwood's Low-Fat Prescription For Kids* (Penguin, 1995).

These changes are far more important for your child and your family than most pediatricians and nutritionists seem to realize. As we've noted several times, on a typical American diet, according to the Bogalusa Heart Study's twenty-five years of reports, fatty deposits are found in the coronary arteries as early as age three. By junior high school age, these fatty deposits are present in over two-thirds of children. The deposits become thicker throughout the teens, and virtually all adults have them by the age of twenty. In contrast, the arteries of vegetarians in this country are clean. Your child's good eating habits depend on you, the parent. Something you can do that will benefit both you and your child is get on with what I call the Family Plan. What are *you* going to eat, while you feed your child a healthier diet? The answer should be obvious: you should make a commitment to eat the same healthy diet yourself. As an adult, you already have some degree of coronary-artery and cancer risk from the diet you've been eating since childhood. The benefits you receive will be more immediate than for your child since you've almost certainly developed some silent heart disease, which may be arrested or even reversed by the Stage 4 diet.

You wouldn't smoke in the presence of your teenager while asking him or her to avoid or give up the habit. Similarly, it becomes extremely awkward to shop for and serve your child Stage 4 foods if other members of the family are still eating a typical high-fat diet.

"I want *Baby and Child Care* to be on the forefront with all this new information we now have at hand," Dr. Spock recently explained to a colleague. His book had already sold nearly fifty million copies—outselling any single book during the twentieth century except the Bible—in forty-two languages. It was time, he thought, to make sure his readers in the year 2000 and beyond had the proper information at hand.

Dr. Spock was right. By the time today's children are adults, it will be common knowledge that the truth was known back in 1998. Parents now have a new responsibility to their children—to prevent heart disease and cancer.

This final edition of Dr. Spock's *Baby and Child Care* was published and shipped to bookstores on May 2, 1998—it would have been his ninety-fifth birthday. He died shortly after finishing the last draft, six weeks earlier, on March 15, 1998. It was his final gift to grateful parents throughout the world.

ASK DR. ATTWOOD

Q : Are most breakfast cereals safe for vegans?

A : Let me give you five criteria to use in choosing breakfast cereals:

- First, choose one that's low-fat (less than 2 grams per serving)
- second, it should be high in fiber (3 grams or more per serving)
- third, it should be low in sugar (less than 3 grams per serving)
- fourth, it should be low in sodium (under 250 mg per serving)
- and fifth, it should be whole grain. Oatmeal and original Cheerios® are good examples.

SEVENTEEN

THE TRUTH ABOUT OLIVE OIL

The "Mediterranean Diet," which seems to be characterized by moderate to large amounts of olive oil and other monounsaturated oils and fats, has gained an increasingly large following among nutritionists and scientists during recent years. The undisputed fact, that the Greeks, Italians, Turks, and especially inhabitants of the Island of Crete, have less coronary heart disease than people in the Western nations, has given olive oil a very good nutritional reputation. So let's take a real hard look. Just how healthy is this mostly monounsaturated oil?

And that's just what it is—a mostly monounsaturated oil. However, it's 100 percent fat, and 16 percent of it is the dreaded saturated fat that clings to our arteries. Studies at the University of South Carolina by Blankenhorn, on humans subjects, and at Bowman Gray School of Medicine by Lawrence Rudel, on monkeys, have shown that this amount of saturated fat is enough to cause new plaques in the coronary arteries and a progression of old lesions in people who already have heart disease.

So why do the Mediterraneans have less heart disease than Americans? The obvious answer is that they ingest relatively less saturated fat than Americans. They've replaced it with the mostly monounsaturated olive oil. But Asians have even less heart disease on a diet of *less total fat* than either Americans or Mediterraneans.

I'm not an olive oil basher. I probably consume it in moderation several times a week. But there are a few troubling caveats: Olive oil crowds out other nutrients, and its 120 calories per tablespoon contains no minerals, no fiber and no vitamins, with the exception of vitamin E. If people are eating excessive amounts of olive oil calories, they're usually eating fewer fruits and vegetables. That means less fiber, zinc and iron.

The researchers who've had the most success with reversal of coronary heart disease, namely Dr. Dean Ornish and Dr. Caldwell Esselstyn, allow no olive oil in their patients' diets. And, by the same token, I would suggest for those people who wish to prevent this disease: Let's go *light* on the olive oil—maybe even lighter than light.

ASK DR. ATTWOOD

Q: I am twenty-four years old, five feet eight inches tall, and weigh around 110-115 pounds. I am interested in a veggie diet and lifestyle, but I am concerned I will lose weight. I am already thin. How can I prevent losing any more weight?

A: You can usually consume as many calories on a vegan diet as you did on a meat- and dairy-based diet. If your weight begins to drop, try adding calories from mostly unsaturated fats, such as nuts, avocados, soy, and you may add some olive oil. Don't overdo this. You should be able to maintain your weight without added oils.

EIGHTEEN

A NEW VEGETARIAN DIET ENDORSEMENT

When my book, *Dr. Attwood's Low-Fat Prescription for Kids* (Penguin) was first published in 1995, it had almost universal acceptance. Parents, grandparents, physicians and educators all seemed to embrace my ideas about vegetarian diets for the whole family. Many members of one professional group, however, seemed uncomfortable with an all plant-based diet. These were the registered dietitians. This was unfortunate, I thought, because they do the greater part of all nutritional counseling in the country. What was wrong?

It seems that many dietitians had not yet been fully informed about the practicality and healthfulness of a vegetarian diet. Many still adhered to the old myth that careful combining of foods was necessary in order to get proper amounts of "complete protein." Others were worried about inadequate calcium, iron and zinc. Still others were concerned about deficiencies of essential fatty acids. In fact, it seemed that the rank-and-file dietition was still operating under the influence of the "Twelve

Common Myths of a Vegetarian Diet" that I wrote about at length in my book.

Encouragingly, there were signs of "vegetarian leadership" among the registered dietitions of the 1990s. The most visible may have been Suzanne Havala and Reed Mangels. Suzanne enjoyed a distinguished professional reputation among the registered dietitions as well as among vegetarians. Reed Mangels, along with Suzanne, is the nutrition co-editor of *Vegetarian Journal*, the official publication of the Vegetarian Resource Group.

The American Dietetic Association (ADA), the professional group to which practically all registered dietitians belong, was also concerned about their members not getting up-to-date information about plant-based nutrition. Enter the latest in a series of opinions on vegetarian diets published by this group. And, it was good news! If you're a vegetarian and you're looking for approval, you've got it. The ADA published its new and updated position paper on vegetarian diets in September 1996. This lifestyle is now considered to be healthy by the most prestigious nutrition association in the U.S.

The ADA's list of life-threatening diseases and disorders found to be reduced among vegetarians includes coronary heart disease, hypertension, obesity, Type 2 diabetes, lung cancer, colorectal cancer, breast cancer and renal disease. This is incredible! They have actually given vegetarians their blessings, almost unconditionally.

Quality proteins of sufficient quantity for good health, they say, may be obtained from a variety of vegetables, whole grains and legumes. All vitamins and minerals, including calcium, may also be obtained from a vegetarian diet, with the exception of vitamin B-12 (see

Chapter 13, page 89) and vitamin D if sun exposure is limited. B-12 supplements or sources should be consumed, the report says, by all persons of any age who eat no animal products, but B-12 absorption, they add, may be diminished as one ages, so they recommend supplements of this vitamin for all older vegetarians and breast-fed infants if the mother's diet is not supplemented.

Finally, the report states that a vegetarian diet is appropriate for all ages, including women during pregnancy and lactation, infants, children, adolescents and teenagers, including athletes. Hopefully, this new ADA position paper will find its way into physician's offices, where, for the most part, there continues to be misunderstanding of vegetarian diets.

The ADA's official position paper on vegetarian diets can be obtained by calling 1-800-877-1600, extension 4896, or by e-mail at hod@eatright.org

ASK DR. ATTWOOD

Q: I'm afraid that I don't get enough fiber from the food I eat. Since my job requires that I travel extensively, I have trouble finding enough fruits and vegetables on the road. As a result, I'm often constipated. What fiber supplements do you recommend?

A: The fiber you need is always more effective when it's obtained from whole foods. First, take a good look at some of the best sources of fiber, both soluble and insoluble, which are effective in preventing constipation. Whole grain breads, pasta, brown rice, fruit and breakfast cereals would be the most easily found while traveling. Vegetables and legumes are great fiber sources, but as you say, not easy to find while traveling. I often grab an apple and a whole-wheat bagel when going through an airport, so I won't have to eat the high-fat low-fiber food usually served on the plane.

There are several sources of supplemental fiber, usually the soluble variety, which may be stirred into a glass of water. Metamucil® and Konsyl-D® (both psyllium husk) and Citrucel® (methyl cellulose) are the most commonly used. However, a more natural supplement of soluble fiber might be adding bran, especially oat bran, to hot cereals or other foods. Remember, fiber works best when extra water is consumed, both by drinking it and by eating fruits and vegetables.

Finally, I like to remind people that no fiber exists in any animal product—none.

PART TWO

CLEARING UP MISINFORMATION

The most dangerous of all falsehoods
is a slightly distorted truth.

—G.C. Lichtenberg,
18th century physicist

NINETEEN

ENTER THE ZONE
A Giant Leap Backwards

Anne, an old friend of mine, walked up to Barry Sears at the Tom Landry Sports Medicine and Research Center in Dallas. She complained that the program outlined in his book, *Enter The Zone*—more lean meat, egg whites, poultry and fish while limiting many grains, vegetables and fruits—just didn't work for her. She didn't feel good, and her performance level while swimming had declined. Anne was now back on her vegetables, fruits and whole grains.

"Stay with what works best," Sears said, "but you know, Anne, it's not the fat and protein that's so important. It's the effect of carbohydrates upon hormones and insulin levels." Though this was contrary to everything I had told Anne about nutrition, the book's message was loud and clear: "All those trendy high-carbohydrate diets," he had written, "may be increasing your risk of developing heart disease." Such nonsense!

Excessive complex carbohydrates, according to Sears, also causes obesity by increasing insulin output and fat storage. This is the process, he insists, that creates bad eicosanoids leading to heart disease and cancer. "To complete a 'Zone-favorable' meal," he advises, "always add fat, the building blocks for eicosanoids."

While it's true that eicosanoids are hormones involved in many metabolic processes, the relation of "bad" eicosanoids to obesity and disease is at best a scientifically unproven gimmick. Unfortunately, however, it has captured the unquestioning reader's imagination.

Every few years since the early 1950s, someone has based a book on carbohydrate bashing. First, there were the *Dr. Stillman's Diet* and *Dr. Atkins' Diet*, followed by *The Scarsdale Diet*, and finally, *Enter The Zone.* Now there are others: Michael and Mary Dan Eases's *Protein Power* and Rachael and Richard Heller's *Health For Life*. And once again *Dr. Atkins New Diet Revolution* is back on the bestseller lists.

According to Bonnie Liebman, at the Center For Science in the Public Interest, it's nothing new. "Miracle diets come and go like hemlines, hair-dos, and celebrity romances." Furthermore, they don't work; and all of them have the potential of raising low-density liproprotein (LDL) levels.

A vegetarian diet, according to Sears, is as far as you can get from The Zone. He ignores the fact that individuals who eat vegetarian diets have far less heart disease and cancer, and tend to be leaner, not fatter. Moreover, most clinical studies conducted during the last half-century, clearly show that a high-protein, high-fat, low-carbohydrate diet leads to higher rates of heart disease, stroke, hypertension, adult onset diabetes and many types of cancer. The relationship of animal fat to cancer is stronger than ever before. According to new studies released by the Environmental Protection Agency, potent carcinogens from industrial wastes, such as dioxin and other chlorinated compounds are known to be concentrated in the animal fat of meat, fish, and dairy products. On the other hand, vegetables, fruits and grains contain only traces of these compounds.

Why is The Zone diet so popular? Its followers defend it vehemently, largely because they find the rapid weight loss irresistible. Like most low-carbohydrate diets, however, a great deal of the weight loss is dehydration. Ordinarily, three grams of water are stored with every gram of carbohydrates in the form of glycogen in the liver and skeletal muscles. When this is sharply limited, the desperate "zonies" think they are losing up to a pound of fat a day. It's also low in calories (about 1,700), causing the unhealthy depletion of lean body mass along with the minimal fat loss.

Without careful monitoring, this type of diet may lead to "ketosis" (an unnatural form of acidosis), which often causes some degree of anorexia and even euphoria. Sears denies that this happens with the amount of carbohydrates he allows. However, Dr. Atkins, another proponent of high-protein, high-fat, low-carbohydrate consumption, considers ketosis to be a useful and necessary state. If ketosis sounds familiar, it's also the result when insulin-dependent diabetics can't metabolize carbohydrates without their insulin injections—a state leading up to diabetic coma.

The Sears diet recommends that one get 30 percent of calories from fat, 30 percent from protein, and 40 percent from carbohydrates. It should be obvious that these are approximately the proportions already consumed in most Western countries, including the United States, where heart disease and cancer are rampant. Furthermore, with such low intakes of complex carbohydrates, it appears that Sears' recommended diet would be deficient in vegetables, fruits and whole grains—and would contain inadequate fiber. Adding insult to injury, this level of protein consumption may promote calcium loss and osteoporosis.

Sears has very little to say about cholesterol levels in his book. He writes, "If cholesterol is such a villain, why does the body make so much of it?" The real heart disease risk, he says, is "hyperinsulinemia and bad ecosinoids." Perhaps he is unaware that practically all published reports indicate just the opposite. His book is riddled with such comments as, ". . . eating fat doesn't make you fat." It cautions that some foods—like potatoes, brown rice, bread, corn, carrots, pasta, bananas, dry breakfast cereals, apple juice and orange juice—may be harmful to your health. Again, nonsense! None of the references cited, backing these conclusions, have ever been published, and the book does not contain a reference section or a bibliography.

At a landmark nutritional debate between vegetarian Dr. John McDougall and Barry Sears at the Bally Hotel in Las Vegas in 1997, The Zone diet and its author were seriously challenged. Among numerous objections, Dr. McDougall asserted that, according to the caloric content of The Zone, Sears, who claims to have stayed on the diet for six years, would have seemingly had to start the diet at a weight of over 600 pounds to reduce to his present weight.

In summary, a half-century of scientific research, first from Ansel Keyes' population studies in the 1950s to T. Colin Campbell's ongoing Cornell-Oxford-China Nutrition project today, has given us a wealth of data supporting the health benefits of carbohydrates. The Zone would be a giant step backward. A little weight loss, which is quickly regained when the diet is no longer tolerated, isn't worth the inevitable long-term health risk.

ASK DR. ATTWOOD

Q: Do you have any comments regarding this study that suggests that a "extra-lean diet" may not help many? I have been on a diet of less than 10 percent fat and less than 15 mg. of cholesterol/day for seven years and have never felt better.

A: There are a scattering of studies suggesting that more fat, not less, is recommend, but these studies are seriously flawed. Your diet sounds excellent.

TWENTY

DIOXIN: IT'S EVEN WORSE THAN WE THOUGHT

We passed through endless miles of pristine mountain forests, hugged at the rugged coastline by an almost cobalt blue Atlantic Ocean. The sky, only a shade lighter, was cloudless. Once again, Judy and I were driving up the Maine coast to the little seaside village of Camden. There, Dr. Benjamin Spock and his wife, Mary Morgan, summer residents of Camden, had asked me to work with them again on revisions for the new edition of *Dr. Spock's Baby and Child Care.* As we drove along this beautiful coast, nothing—as far as our eyes could see— would intimate the concern of a newly organized group of Maine citizens, The Dioxin Coalition. This band of environmentalists, public advocates and business leaders were concerned that dioxin, an industrial byproduct, was posing a new and serious health risk to the citizens of their state.

The earliest work on dioxin, done by my friend and colleague Dr. T. Colin Campbell in 1963, identified it as one of the most powerful toxins on earth—an ingredient of the Agent Orange used in Vietnam to defoliate forests. It wasn't until 1994 that the Environmental Protection Agency (EPA) took a serious look at this chlorinated compound. In a 2,000-page document, the EPA stated that this waste product of such industrial processes as paper-bleaching and the burning of plastics, was not only a toxin, but also a probable carcinogen similar to formaldehyde and chloroform.

According to the EPA report, dioxin has almost certainly been accumulating for years in the tissues of fish and larger animals. Accordingly, it is present in the tissues of nearly every American who consumes animal-based foods.

As expected, dioxin is concentrated most heavily in larger animals, and once there, it's usually permanent, not readily detoxified or excreted by metabolic processes. Moreover, continued exposures lead to more absorption. One of the few ways dioxin is released from the body—other than prolonged fasting—seems to be through lactation.

Consequently, another source of this compound is the milk of cows, who eat dioxin-contaminated grass, weeds and grains. And if a mother is breastfeeding, stored dioxins are to some degree released to her child. These amounts in breastmilk are likely very small, probably with little risk, but those obtained by eating red meat, fish and dairy products is significant and additive. Obviously, people eating fish from a river where a paper mill discharges water are probably at even greater risk.

Maine, the Coalition says, is a good study model, since it is the second largest paper-producing state, and it burns 30 percent more household trash than other states. Not unexpectedly, trash and medical incinerators have been shown to emit ash heavily laced with dioxin.

Interestingly, dioxin, along with other manufactured, heavily-chlorinated chemicals—polychlorinated bifenals (PCB) and dichlorodiphenyl trichloroethane (DDT)— have an estrogen-like effect upon tissues. This may explain at least one of the mechanisms of the apparent relationship of animal-based foods to the hormone-dependent cancers of the breast, prostate and testes in industrialized Western countries.

But just how important is dioxin as a carcinogen? Animal fat and animal protein, without any industrial contaminants, apparently cause cancer. In the rural areas of China, sharp differences in cancer incidence are found between villagers consuming low and high animal fat and protein diets, where no known industrial pollutants exist. I suspect that natural animal protein and fat account for the greatest majority of food-related cancers. Dr. Campbell agrees. "In my view," he wrote in December 1995, in his editorial for the newsletter *New Century Nutrition,* ". . . no chemical carcinogen is nearly so important in causing human cancer as animal protein."

Dioxin is everything we thought it was, and probably much more. As a toxin it may lead to neuropathies, muscle weakness and even paralysis. As a carcinogen, it's much more subtle and poorly understood. With very few pathways of detoxification or excretion, its effects are almost certainly cumulative and in most cases permanent. While it's uncertain how much dioxin one can tolerated without serious consequences, it's obvious that this compound should be avoided wherever possible.

Many of my patients have become alarmed after reading newspaper accounts about dioxin. But escaping the slow and progressive absorption of this chemical, as it turns out, is far simpler than most would have expected. Dr. Beverly Pagan, senior staff scientist at Jackson Laboratories in Bar Harbor, Maine, reminds us that dioxin cannot be absorbed by inhalation from the air, and so can be avoided if people eat low on the food chain. "Those who follow a vegetarian diet," she says, "usually don't have to worry about dioxin."

Vegetables, fruits and grains do not contain concentrated amounts of this compound. This fact, along with the thousands of cancer-inhibiting phytochemicals in these foods, all working in concert, once again reminds us that human nutrition is really not that complex. A plant-based diet of whole foods does it all for us. Calories, grams of fat, grams of protein, vitamins, minerals, phytochemicals and antioxidants are all there in the right amounts and working their magic. The only things missing or deficient are animal fat, protein and, of course, dioxin.

ASK DR. ATTWOOD

Q: I read the article on your website about dioxin with great interest. I have had tremendous, unfocused fear about this pollutant for a long time, and what you had to say allayed a lot of my worries.

My question is, if it's so hard for a vegetarian human to absorb dangerous amounts of dioxin on a diet of plant sources, why do our herbivore cousins, the cows, absorb enough to become themselves a dioxin risk? I have been a vegetarian for many years, and the news that my chosen lifestyle benefits me by keeping dioxin out of my diet is thrilling to hear! Still, something in the logic seems to be missing for me. If you can shed any light on this misunderstanding I would appreciate it.

A: Large animals such as cattle get dioxin directly from downstream pollution of burning plastics and paper mills. The state of Maine, for instance, contains much of this—therefore, the existence of Maine's Coalition Group. Also, pollution from the burning plastics, etc., after being ingested in water and grass by cattle is concentrated within the cattle liver. It's excreted in concentrated form in their milk.

Washed fruits and vegetables do not contain concentrated dioxin as dioxin contains no binders and can be washed off the outside of these foods. Always wash your fruits and vegetables before eating them. You're doing just fine. Keep up the good work.

TWENTY-ONE

THE GERBER
CONTROVERSY

The young mother had no idea that the jar of baby food she had just given her infant wasn't all fruit. Nothing on the label had shown that the bananas were only 50 percent of the feeding. The rest was added water, sugar and modified starch (which has been given the name, Tapioca). The product—not only this jar of bananas, but dozens of other fruits and vegetables sold by Gerber, a brand widely advertised as being recommended by four out of five pediatricians—has dominated the shelf-space in food stores for decades. Comparable foods manufactured by Beech-Nut, Earth's Best and even Gerber's own first-stage products—those suggested for infants under six months of age—contain 100 percent fruits or vegetables.

According to the Center for Science in the Public Interest (CSPI), this unbelievable "baby-cheating" practice had been the standard at Gerber for several generations, but the company had consistently reassured both parents and pediatricians that its products were the most nutritious money could buy. As for the claim that Gerber baby foods were recommended by four out of five pediatricians, CSPI found that the survey quoted showed something else entirely. Only one in five pediatricians recommended any specific brand of baby food. Of those who did, four of five recommended Gerber. But overall, only about 16 percent of pediatricians recommended Gerber. The company has consistently failed to make this clear, despite persistent complaints to the Federal Trade Commission.

Since whole fruits and vegetables are children's principal sources for thousands of phytochemicals, both known and unknown—all of which necessarily work together to prevent chronic degenerative diseases, such as heart disease and many cancers—it seems important that consumers know when they are getting whole, not diluted, foods. Fiber, both soluble and insoluble, is another important ingredient that is greatly diminished in these diluted products.

The ingredient section of the label should show percentages of the primary foods contained in the jars, but Gerber has resisted this for many years. The obvious reason in my opinion is that diluted food can be sold for less, thereby allowing Gerber to undersell the competition. This is not the reason given by Gerber. They've insisted that it was done to enhance taste. Yet, babies have found other undiluted brands and homemade baby food from a blender just as tasty.

Heinz, the second-largest producer of baby foods is less expensive, according to *Consumer Reports* in their September 1996 issue, and "just as nutritious." (That's because, says the CSPI, they contain "relatively little food.") The *Consumer Report* fails to tell the reader that the Heinz counterpart of Gerber's *Bananas with Tapioca* is only about 25 percent bananas. And, like Gerber, many of Heinz's other products also contain large amounts of fillers.

In January 1996, CSPI's director Michael Jacobson and I co-signed a letter to 20,000 pediatricians, pointing out this dilution of baby foods, using the Gerber banana product as an example. We followed this with a national press conference in Washington.

Gerber's response to this was simply that their product was the industry leader. However, within a few weeks the FDA had received an unprecedented 1500 letters from pediatricians throughout the country, all expressing their concern for the Gerber practice of diluting baby foods.

Gerber still insisted that the added modified starch and sugar were necessary to enhance the taste. But surprisingly, a short time later, the CSPI was notified that the company would no longer be diluting their second- and third-stage fruits and vegetables. Their new labels: 100% Fruit; or 100% Vegetables.

Why this sudden change? According to CSPI, *Advertising Age* magazine had reported that Gerber's share of the U.S. market had dropped from 80 percent to 65 percent during the few months following our press conference. And a short time later, six class-action suits were filed against the company for misleading advertising. Not unexpectedly, within the next few weeks Heinz announced similar changes.

Also the "four out of five pediatricians" claim will probably be discontinued, since it was considered misleading by the Federal Trade Commission.

According to the CSPI, "We have won!" I agreed. A giant company—Gerber is a division of Sandoz—had taken a first step to a more healthful and honest policy, despite the obvious cost. I found this even more significant when I realized that baby food isn't for babies alone. It's also used regularly to sustain the nutritional needs of thousands of older individuals.

Gerber spokesperson Barbara Ivans admits that their baby food is often used by the elderly, either in nursing homes or by both the elderly and disabled who are cared for at home. According to Neva Linscombe, director of the Landmark Nursing Home in Crowley, Louisiana, despite it's greater expense, elderly and disabled adults seem to prefer the taste over that of pureed food prepared by institutions. What they prefer, apparently, is the "enhanced" Gerber taste accomplished by the sugar and starch fillers. Already at high risk for heart disease, cancer and constipation, these individuals especially need the nutrients and fiber of whole foods.

The real issue here was the continued inadequate labeling requirements of the FDA, despite its greatly improved revisions mandated by the Nutrition Labeling and Education Act of 1990. The new labels, which appeared in May 1994, still failed to reveal the ingredient amounts. If a list of main ingredients had also included the ingredients' percentages, there would have been no Gerber or Heinz problem. But presently, whether the consumer is concerned about whole-food ingredients or something detrimental to their health, such as hydrogenated oils, they have no way of knowing how much is present. So far, unfortunately, the FDA has remained clearly on the side of the food processors.

ASK DR. ATTWOOD

Q: Although I'm still breast-feeding my baby and plan to for as long as possible, I have begun feeding my eight-month-old a natural, processed baby food. I would like to start making baby food myself, but I'm not quite sure how to do it and what I should be feeding my child. Any suggestions?

A: I commend you for your commitment to breast-feeding your baby for as long as possible. However, even the best processed baby food is just pureed vegetables. You can do the same thing with a food processor or by mashing the food yourself. Fruits, vegetables, legumes and grains should be pureed or mashed as needed, and introduced in that order. These form the basis of an ideal diet at any age, although your family may wish to include other foods as well. Children under two will be getting additional needed fat from mother's milk (or formula), and some richer foods of your choice, such as avocado (mashed alone or with banana), or full-fat tofu (good pureed with a green vegetable). For more information on infant feeding, I recommend *The Womanly Art of Breast-feeding* from La Leche League International, or *Pregnancy, Children, and the Vegan Diet* by Michael Klaper, M.D.

TWENTY-TWO

THE GREAT OLESTRA BLUNDER

How Did it Happen?

The last meeting of the FDA's Food Advisory Committee (FAC) was underway at a Holiday Inn in Alexandria, Virginia. Twenty-three experts from universities and research centers throughout the country had met there the previous three days for working sessions. It was November 17, 1995 and they would be making a decision about whether or not to recommend that the FDA approve Proctor & Gamble's new fat substitute, *olestra*. It was a cloudy, chilly day in Washington, but this FAC meeting was especially well attended by both working members of the committee and other invited experts. Their sole objective, they were reminded repeatedly by FDA Commissioner, Dr. David Kessler, who was there the last two days, would be a "reasonable certainty of no harm" from this product. "That is not the same thing," he told them, "as concluding that it is not dangerous."

Olestra had been under development for twenty-five years at a total cost of over $200 million. It had all the qualities of fat, but wasn't absorbed and therefore left behind no calories and no fat. It was heat-stable and could be used for both frying and baking. But there were caveats. Dr. Fred H. Mattson, the co-discoverer and former employee of P&G—now with the University of California—said later in an interview for *TIME Magazine* about his work on the product, "We had a great deal of trouble with what we called 'anal leakage.'" It seems that in some individuals this new substance, a sucrose molecule, a polyester, with six to eight long-chain fatty acids attached, was so large and dense that enzymes couldn't break it down. It went through the gastrointestinal tract without absorption and actually stained the underwear of test subjects. Though this risk of "anal leakage" and underwear staining has been reduced, according to researchers at P&G, by making changes or "stiffening" the molecule, it hasn't been abolished. The final product continued to cause bloating, cramping and diarrhea in many individuals eating as little as the 10 grams contained in a small, one-ounce bag of potato chips. There is also evidence that this effect is greater in patients with chronic inflammatory bowel disease.

Other problems discussed by the Food Advisory Committee were the disturbing findings by P&G that fat soluble vitamins A, D, E, and K apparently attached themselves to this large fatty-acid polyester molecule and were carried out with it instead of being absorbed. Several subgroups may be at high risk, such as persons on anticoagulant medication, children, the elderly, pregnant women and persons with chronic inflammatory bowel disease; none of these groups had been adequately studied.

Olestra also interfered with the absorption of

carotenoids, some of which are also fat-soluble. The long-term effects of carotenoid depletion is unknown, but most experts studying this nutrient fear an increased cancer risk to be the result. There has also been a link between carotenoid deficiencies and macular degeneration, which results in permanent blindness among the elderly.

One study conducted in Holland and reported in the *American Journal of Clinical Nutrition* (62:591, 1995) showed that after one month of eating just 3 grams of olestra daily (an amount contained in only six potato chips), the blood levels of lycopene (a carotenoid found in tomatoes, and suspected of preventing prostate cancer), was 40 percent less than in controls who didn't eat olestra-containing foods.

The committee suggested that products made with olestra should have added fat-soluble vitamins to counteract their concurrent depletion. However, they felt that carotenoids had not been proven to be of value in preventing cancer or other disorders.

Unlike the cramps and diarrhea, consumers cannot monitor the long-term risk of carotenoid depletion. Yet, some members of the FAO suggested that the public will "vote at the cash register."

Among the members of the Food Advisory Committee who strongly urged the approval of olestra from the beginning was Dr. Ronald Kleinman, a Harvard pediatrician and frequent spokesman for the American Academy of Pediatrics. During the committee meetings on November 16 and 17, according to internal FDA documents, he acknowledged the fact that children eating food containing this substance may have cramping or diarrhea. If children get sick from it, he suggested, they can stop eating olestra containing foods. "They may not wish to tolerate four or five bowel movements a day, but I don't see that that has an adverse effect on their health if they stop that food. I don't believe I am hard-hearted."

Another member of the committee, Dr. Henry Blackburn of the University of Minnesota, seemed to have strong reservations about this product throughout the discussions. Later, he would say, "...it appears that to prevent approval, there would have to be absolute proof that a food additive is harmful. It shifts the burden of proof from the company to the public." He also complained that several committee members have worked as consultants to the food industry. He later repeated these concerns in an editorial for the *New England Journal of Medicine.*

When the November 17th meeting ended, three members didn't vote, citing a conflict of interest; five voted against approval, and fifteen voted for approval for use in salty snacks, potato chips, corn chips and crackers, with the following warning displayed on the package: "This product contains olestra. Olestra may cause abdominal cramping and loose stools. Olestra inhibits the absorption of some vitamins and other nutrients. Vitamins A, D, E, and K have been added."

The words diarrhea or anal leakage were not recommended, and no mention was made about the inhibition of carotenoid absorption.

During the time between the committee's adjournment on November 19th and the December 1st deadline for public comments—a deadline that was later extended—nearly 800 letters poured into the Rockville,

146

Maryland, Dockets Management Branch of the FDA. Most letters, according to *New York Times* food columnist Marion Burros, were from nutritionists and scientists recommending that the product not be approved. Strong objections were spearheaded by the Washington, D.C.-based consumer advocacy group, Center for Science in the Public Interest, led by Dr. Michael Jacobson. The American Public Health Association, the American Academy of Ophthalmology, the Lifestyle Medicine Institute and the National Women's Health Network all came out against approval.

Several well-known nutritionists sent letters recommending rejection, including Dr. Marian Nestle, NYU's chief nutritionist. Dr. Walter Willett and Meir Stampfer of the Harvard School of Public Health wrote to Commissioner Kessler: ". . . the fact that P&G wishes to proceed with the introduction of olestra into U.S. diets is appalling . . . over fifty studies have found, with remarkable consistency, that diets rich in carotenoids are associated with lower risk of cancer at many sites." But the decision was now totally up to Commissioner Kessler.

Meanwhile, P&G—who, according to former employees, had been prepared to spend another $800 million if necessary to get this potential $1-billion-a-year product on the market—was apparently becoming concerned by this influx of new mail to the FDA. They would take no chances. Victory, it seemed, was near.

On December 15th, P&G asked dozens of scientists to write letters to the FDA on its behalf. They were actually given a guideline of points to make, including (1) your area of expertise, (2) olestra's general or G.I. (gastrointestinal) safety or benefit, (3) reasonable certainty of no harm, with a recommendation that the FDA should approve it, (4) the carotenoid and G.I. effects have been fully addressed by the FDA's Food Advisory Committee, (5) olestra's health benefits, and (6) commend the FDA on its thorough process. Of the twenty-six scientists who complied with P&G's request and wrote letters to the FDA urging approval of the product, some were or had been consultants to P&G, others had been a part of the FDA Food Advisory Committee, and still others had attended the public committee meeting on November 17th.

On January 25, 1996, olestra was approved for marketing. Five days later a copy of the required warning label was filed in the Federal Register, still with no mention of the words diarrhea or carotenoids.

Test marketing of olestra by Frito-Lay company in their Max potato chips began in April '96 in three cities— Cedar Rapids, Iowa; Eau Clair, Wisconsin and Grand Junction, Colorado. The product went nationwide in 1998 under the brand name, WOW. P&G's own Pringles potato chips, prepared with the new product, soon followed.

So, is it all over? Not exactly. The FDA approval of olestra was based on a required ongoing study of side effects by the company, which was reviewed by the same FAC in June, 1998.

Proctor & Gamble next asked for approval to market olestra, despite a number of disappointing taste tests, under the brand name Olean, to all food companies for use in hundreds, even thousands of products. Already the giant leap had been made from laboratory animals (pigs), to 250 million human test subjects. Now, the real answer to the question about the safety of olestra will depend on how many new cases of heart disease, cancer and blindness develop in those who consume it. This may not be known for many years.

What is the typical consumer saying? As I travel and speak, I find most people highly suspicious of olestra, but not without humor. In Kalamazoo, Michigan a college student said, "Why don't they market it as a laxative?" Another mused, "Proctor & Gamble makes this food product that causes anal leakage. They also make a laundry detergent."

ASK DR. ATTWOOD

Q: I recently read that Proctor and Gamble received government approval to use Olestra/Olean in a wide variety of products. Does this mean that it's safe and there are no more concerns about eating foods that contain it? I have seen the advertising that claims that Olean makes snacks "a little healthier," and Frito-Lay says that their Wow chips are "safe" for everyone."

A: According to the Center for Science in the Public Interest (a nonprofit health-advocacy organization) : "*The New England Journal of Medicine* is not allowing a deceptive Olean ad to run again. It is a decision others should emulate."

Although the advertising may not say it, the labels still do. In part, the government-required labeling says, "Olestra may cause abdominal cramping and loose stools." As we have seen in the past, the government will give approval to items that later prove to be unsafe. I would not suggest eating any products that contains Olestra.

If you want a fat-free chip (and Olestra is not fat-free), I would suggest that you buy baked chips, which actually are fat free, and which do not have the same health risks assoicated with them that Olestra/Olean products do.

A VEGETARIAN DOCTOR SPEAKS OUT

TWENTY-THREE

The Worst Scientific Report Ever

*Truth is the most valuable thing we have,
let us encourage it.*
—Mark Twain (1835-1910)

Newspapers all over the world reprinted the story reported in a study published by the *Journal of the American Medical Association* in the fall of 1997. The study, part of the world famous, ongoing Framingham Heart Study, strongly suggested that eating a high-fat diet prevented strokes in a group of 832 healthy middle-aged men.

Beginning in the late 1960s, the subjects were asked one time to recall what they had eaten during the previous twenty-four hours. During the following twenty years, the men who had reported the highest fat intake had fewer ischemic strokes, the common type produced by a blockage of the arteries supplying the brain.

It should have been clear to the researchers that they couldn't reach any kind of conclusion over a twenty-year period based on a single twenty-four-hour food intake recall. However, the study was published in the prestigious *JAMA*, and as a result, reported shamelessly by the media around the world.

All other evidence from studies over the past half-century would have led us to believe just the opposite—that less fat would reduce the risk of stroke. But the word was out and, once again, the general public—who desperately needed accurate and consistent information—was hopelessly confused. Worse yet, thousands may have discounted the value of a low-fat diet, and would now be a higher risk for both heart disease and stroke.

Just when I was beginning to think that this kind of news media confusion had begun to subside, an elderly gentlemen walked up to me after my nutrition lecture in Wichita, Kansas. He said, "Doctor, according to this publication you are all wrong about fat." Then he showed me the same story in the current issue of the AARP newspaper avidly read by millions of elderly people.

A single, flawed, but widely-touted study, had created an overwhelming and misleading effect upon the very people who depend upon their medical authorities for guidance. People who had been struggling with their "fat-taste" would now be more confused than ever. Many would now undoubtedly resume their poor eating habits.

ASK DR. ATTWOOD

Q: I am a very fit individual. I just received results of a blood test and my triglyceride level was 384, while my glucose was a mere 1. These results are mg./dl. Also my HDL was 40 mg./dl and LDL was 61 mg./dl. Cholesterol was 170.

I tend to get hungry and usually eat every two-to-three hours, otherwise I get tired. I crave sweets all the time but eat a diet including a large amount of fruits and vegetables. What advice can you give me to reduce my triglycerides to a normal level? Also what are the risks of having such high levels?

A: I would repeat these tests after fasting for twelve hours. High triglyceride levels such as yours may be nothing more that excessive consumption of simple sugars and lots of fruit. Your cholesterol and HDL were okay, but the high triglyceride level could throw off the value of your LDL, since the calculation required a fasting triglyceride value. LDL= Cholesterol (minus) (HDL + one-fifth of triglycerides).

TWENTY-FOUR

VEGETARIAN FAMILIES AND THE COURTS

Social workers from the California Department of Children's Services (DCS) arrived at the McBride School for handicapped children in Los Angeles shortly before noon on September 20, 1995. They took five-year-old Monea Hromadko from her classroom to nearby Cedars-Sinai Medical Center, according to her father, without his knowledge. Peter Hromadko, a single parent, said he was shocked when he learned later that evening that she would not be coming home; the state was taking his daughter from him because he and Monea were vegetarians.

It all started a few days earlier, when the school nurse, concerned about Monea's small stature, poor growth, and speech delays—she had a congenital neurological disorder—noted that the child and her father were vegetarians who consumed no meat or dairy products. The nurse had misunderstood Peter's suggestion to offer his daughter fruit if she wouldn't eat other food at school, and reported to DCS that Monea ate only fruit.

Monea was rarely sick, but had been diagnosed with developmental problems since birth.

At Cedars, assuming that her small statue was due to malnutrition, specific written instructions were given for more protein, including meat, cheese, cream cheese, sour cream, beef, hotdogs, gravy, peanut butter and milk. It was suggested that fresh fruits and vegetables be limited, because they were too bulky. The State of California, however, quickly removed Monea from the custody of her father, despite his pleadings.

It was then that I was contacted by Dr. James DeAndrea, a Los Angeles physician who had taken a special interest in the case. He asked, on the father's behalf, for my help in preparing for the upcoming hearing before the judge. "Could I," Dr. DeAndrea asked, "supply material about vegetarian diets for children?" Adding, "We must stop this." Dr. DeAndrea was concerned about the state establishing such a precedent.

After being assured by Dr. DeAndrea that I had all the facts, I sent material from my book, *Dr. Attwoods's Low-Fat Prescription For Kids* (Penguin, 1995), from columns in New Century Nutrition by Dr. Benjamin Spock and myself, and secured a copy of the American Dietetic Association's (ADA) "Position Paper on Vegetarian Diets" written by Suzanne Havala.

And it worked! Dr. DeAndrea prepared a presentation for the judge, using the material we sent, and Monea was finally returned to the custody of her father on December 18, 1995. Later, on January 20, 1996, all charges by the state were officially dropped. Since then there have been no further state objections to the vegetarian diet of the Hromadko family. Was this incidence a rare occurrence?

Maybe not. What I know is that some vegetarian families haven't fared as well.

Shirley Dumas and her husband James, of Gary, Indiana, were told that state welfare agents had come to their church looking for them on January 23, 1996. Later that day, at about 8:30 P.M., there was a knock at the door of their home. There, Shirley was confronted by two members of Child Protective Services (CPS), a social welfare agency of the State of Indiana, and two armed policemen. They insisted, she said, that she strip the clothing from Jeremiah, the seventeenth-month-old son she and James had adopted eight months earlier. They inspected the child for bruises and then asked if they could look in the refrigerator.

Shirley reports that when she said "No," and demanded to know what this was all about, the refrigerator was opened anyway. She was then told that their son was being taken into state custody because she and James were not feeding him proper food. The refrigerator search was done, they told her, to confirm that there was no meat in the house. It was known at CPS that the Shirley and James were vegetarians.

Decidedly, Jeremiah was small for his age, but Shirley, who has a degree in early childhood education, had known at the time of the adoption that he likely had fetal alcohol effects and would grow more slowly than a normal infant. To assure that Jeremiah was properly fed she had regularly read about nutrition and sought advice from health-food stores. His meals consisted of a varied diet of vegetables, fruits, legumes and goat's milk. He especially likes lentils. When she explained this to the agents from CPS, their only response was that they were only doing their jobs.

The vegetarian practices of the Dumas family began shortly after they were married, ten years ago. When they met, James was interested in herbs and Shirley was already reading about the health benefits of plant-based food. "So it was just natural that we became vegetarians," Shirley said.

Shirley and James Dumas had another disadvantage not shared by Peter Hromadko. It actually resulted, she thinks, from their interest in handicapped children, especially those born to mothers who abused drugs or alcohol. They had been foster parents until two years ago when the state discovered that they were vegetarians. At the time, they were caring for three children, including a developmentally-handicapped child who was severely premature at birth. Their foster-parent license was revoked. They complained bitterly at the state level, which now, they admit, may have tarnished their images as parents. "Now they were watching us when we adopted Jeremiah."

The Hromadko and Dumas cases are presented here not to frighten vegetarian families, but to illustrate the issue, and to offer a means by which parents can gather authoritative information in defense of their vegetarian lifestyles. It's a scenario that I'm beginning to see more and more often. Admittedly, I've heard only one side of the Dumas story—the state agency will not discuss the case with either me or others who have inquired. Merritt Clifton, a second-generation vegetarian and editor of *Animal People*, a monthly animal rights newspaper—who also has an extensive background in child protection services—is withholding judgement. He feels that more information is needed in order to conclude that these families weren't negligent.

Since this case came to my attention in early March 1996, I've reviewed dozens of documents supplied to me by the Dumas family, including Jeremiah's medical records, growth charts, documents about his probable fetal alcohol effects, character references from neighbors and an employee at the Indiana Family and Social Services Administration, and Shirley's early child education certificate. But most of all, I've talked at length with Shirley several times. She is, in my opinion, knowledgeable about a proper plant-based diet. She says that she and James are devastated, as all their early bonding, she worries, may be lost. Ironically, based on all the facts I have, Jeremiah was probably on a more healthful diet than most of his peers. Once again, I'll send documents for the judge, including my book, the ADA's position paper, Dr. Spock's diet recommendations in *New Century Nutrition,* and my strong opinion.

Like Merritt Clifton, I also have an extensive background in child protection services. Since 1964, as a practicing pediatrician I've served as the primary physician with my community's Child Protection Agency. Some days I'm asked as many as five times to evaluate children for alleged neglect or abuse. These investigations have usually been initiated by an anonymous complaint by a neighbor, a friend, or even a relative. I've found no neglect or abuse in the majority of these; but whatever I report, it's the agency and a judge who make the decision about whether or not to remove a child from his or her parents.

Are vegetarian families at risk from well-meaning but

improperly educated social workers and judges? These people have enormous power, but in most cases their knowledge of nutrition is lacking. A family may be disrupted forever, depending upon their suspicions.

Could this be the tip of an iceberg? I wonder. Since I've become involved in the Hromadko and Dumas cases, several other vegetarian families have contacted me concerning state agency threats of taking their children, and even court orders to feed them meat and milk. Unfortunately, social workers and judges learned about food in grade school—just like the rest of us—from materials and advertising supplied by the National Dairy Council and the National Beef Industry Council. If this must be accepted in order to live in a free country, then we must also accept the possibility that innocent parents are sometimes fallaciously accused of child neglect. Shirley's response to this during one of our interviews was: "But this is America!" But her son, Jeremiah was never returned.

If you should ever have to justify the vegetarian lifestyle of your child to a state agency or a judge, their concern will generally be about his or her growth. You should go to the hearing with the documents described below. Their detailed references are found in *Dr. Attwood's Low-Fat Prescription for Kids* (Penguin,1995).

1. One of the most authoritative reports is a review of all available scientific studies by the Department of Family Medicine at the University of California at San Diego in 1992. Their conclusion was that a vegetarian diet is perfectly compatible with normal growth when adequate calories are consumed.

2. Normal growth among vegetarian Seventh Day Adventist school children compared to those in public schools was reported by Loma Linda University in 1991. Ironically, the Adventist children attained a greater adult height.

3. A Federal survey by the CDC of 404 vegetarian children, commonly known as The Farm Study, was done in a rural Tennessee planned community in 1989. Their report in *Pediatrics* found their growth to be normal.

This much we know: Vegetarian children who receive adequate calories grow more slowly during their teens than children consuming animal products, but reach full adult height. And finally, heart disease and cancer of the breast, prostate and colon are far less common among adults who grew up as vegetarian children.

ASK DR. ATTWOOD

Q: Our family stopped eating meat, poultry, fish and dairy products several years ago. We're confirmed vegetarians. Often when we invite guests for lunch or dinner, I feel slightly embarrassed not offering them more typical food that they are used to. On the other hand, I can't bear to cook food that I feel is so unhealthy. Any suggestions?

A: Don't apologize for your commitment to a healthy plant-based diet. I share your strong opinion about meat and dairy products. You wouldn't offer them cigarettes if they were smokers.

My friend, the late Dr. Spock, and his wife, Mary Morgan once invited me, along with several others who weren't vegetarians, to their Maine home to work on book revisions. When they arrived we drove everyone to the local farmer's market, giving each guest a wicker basket and a twenty-dollar bill. Each was given the job of shopping for a variety of vegetables, fruit and bread. We cooked this on the deck while the book revisions progressed throughout the day. Everyone enjoyed it immensely.

TWENTY-FIVE

"IT'S A QUALITY OF LIFE ISSUE!"

For years, the argument some people have made about smoking has been: "It's a quality of life issue!" The logic went like this: "I love smoking. Maybe it's not so good for me, but so what? At least I'll be happy. At least I'll enjoy myself more. At least I'll die happy!" But fewer people are saying this anymore because they've seen the long-term effects of smoking: lung cancer, emphysema, stroke, etc. And they really would like to live longer, be with their friends and family longer, and avoid pushing around an oxygen tank during the final years of their lives.

Today, however, some people are making the same justifications for eating a meal heavily laden with saturated fat and cholesterol. They seem to be looking for excuses to continue an eating style that they know compromises their health. From time to time their excuses are supported by references from the scientific community, which conveniently appear. One such myth that has made the rounds of late, especially among physicians, is the notion that even if all coronary heart disease were

165

prevented, the average individual's life-span would only increase by a matter of months. The media loves to jump on such "studies," but the result can be many confused and discouraged people who have been trying to eat a healthy diet. Some physicians may even begin exhorting their sick patients to "relax and enjoy" themselves.

The unfortunate impact of this kind of misinformation is that many physicians phase out their already meager efforts at reducing their patient's dietary fat. "Now maybe everyone will quit bugging us about cholesterol," is a sentiment that I've heard voiced among physicians in recent hospital staff meetings. The irony is that the general public has always taken the risk of dietary fat far more seriously than have their doctors. A study conducted and published in 1989 revealed the incredible fact that more laypeople than physicians believed that saturated fat and elevated cholesterol levels caused coronary heart disease.

One better-known advocate of the "it's-a-quality-of-life-issue-so-I'll-keep-eating-it" notion was the renowned physician-writer, the late Dr. William Nolan, author of the best seller, *The Making of a Surgeon*. In his final book, *Crisis Time*, Dr. Nolan advised that we should not worry about changing bad habits in order to live a few months longer. Specifically, he pointed to diet, weight control and smoking as acceptable risks.

"If you love rich desserts," he wrote, "even if it raises the likelihood of your dying a year earlier than you would otherwise, by one percent, it's worth it to you." Dr. Nolan, who had already had his second coronary bypass when he wrote this, died a few months later of a massive coronary at the age of fifty-nine.

The unfortunate study that Dr. Nolan and others

focused upon in order to rationalize unhealthy eating patterns was published in a leading medical journal, which is read by most practicing physicians. By eliminating heart disease deaths from the population study, it found that the average life-expectancy increased only slightly in the general population. Of course, the flaw in the study was that it took into account deaths from all causes, such as automobile and other accidents, crime, shootings, cancer, suicide, infant mortality, etc. The study did a huge disservice by failing to point out that those individuals who would have died prematurely of coronary heart disease would, in fact, have had their lives extended *much longer* that just several months.

A 1980 study done among 7,000 residents of Alameda County, California, reported that people with a certain group of lifestyle patterns lived an average of eleven years longer than the general population. The people living longer were nonsmokers, of normal weight, with a moderate alcohol intake, who exercised moderately, ate regular meals and slept seven or eight hours a night.

Studies of Seventh Day Adventists, many of whom are vegetarian, show that their lifestyle—which includes not smoking and using no alcoholic beverages—extends their life span by approximately ten years beyond that of the general population.

By rather moderate health practices, these subjects in the Alameda and the Seventh Day Adventist studies achieved significant gains in life span. Studies noted by the U.S. Department of Health and Human Services and the Department of Agriculture have shown that the consumption of saturated fat is more strongly correlated with mortality than stress or even cigarette smoking. [U.S. Department of Health and Human Services; Department of Agriculture, "The Relationship Between Dietary Cholesterol and Blood Cholesterol."] So, if cholesterol and obesity were successfully controlled—by proper reductions of dietary fat and by increasing dietary fiber by eating primarily vegetables, fruits, whole grains and legumes—consider how much longer one's life span could be extended. Consider, too, what the quality of those extra years would mean to an individual. It's not only about living fifteen more years so you can see your grandchild or great-grandchild graduate from college, it's also about living your final years with vitality, rather than lethargy or illness.

There is, in fact, an overwhelming body of scientific evidence demonstrating an urgent need for reducing dietary fat and protein, and increasing fiber, antioxidants and phytochemicals by consuming plant-based food. Despite this evidence, though, well-meaning writers continue to publish in major medical journals arguments for keeping Americans on their typical, high-fat, high-cholesterol diets. Even the American Heart Association and the National Institutes of Health suggest that our dietary goal should be to consume no more than 30 percent of calories from fat. By eating this way, though, coronary heart disease, stroke, and fat-related cancer will still account for a least half of all adult deaths.

It is perhaps unfortunate—but not surprising—that medical and health institutions are slow to embrace sound dietary measures. In the June 1992 issue of the *Journal of the American College of Nutrition*, the following conclusion was printed: "Moderation is the theme for adequate nutrition." However, "moderation" has proven to be deadly. Studies tell us that people eating a plant-based diet average total serum cholesterol levels of 150.8 mg/dl. [F. Carlson, M. Kipps, A. Lockie and J. Thomas, "A comparative evaluation of vegan, vegetarian and omnivore diets." *Journal of Plant Foods.* 1985;6:89-100.] The Framingham Heart Study has shown conclusively that coronary heart disease vanishes at cholesterol levels below 150 mg/dl. [W. Castelli, "Epidemiology of coronary heart disease: the Framingham study." *Am J Med* 1984; 76(2A);4]. Does the American medical establishment, therefore, advise us to eat a plant-based diet to avoid heart disease? No; they suggest "moderation." But know that the "moderate" American medical establishment considers any level of cholesterol below 200 mg/dl. as "normal." And yes, it is "normal" in a population dying of coronary heart disease at the rate of 978,500 annually. [Science Service, Inc. *Science News* 1989;135 Jan 28. ISSN 0036-8423.]

This book is written for you, not your physician. But I strongly advise you to pass along this information to your doctors. They will not have learned about it in medical school and, with rare exceptions, they won't have shown an interest in it later during their careers. When important advances were made in the control of smoking, *people learned first,* and then taught their doctors. The tobacco industry did not lead the way in pointing out the dangers of smoking. Why would they? We are now concerned with the food industry much like we were forty years ago with the tobacco companies.

On public health issues, physicians must learn from their patients. I call this the "trickle up" effect.

ASK DR. ATTWOOD

Q : We are implementing your plan when we eat at home, but sometimes it's hard when going out. Do you have any tips for healthy eating when dining in restaurants?

A : Dr. Michael DeBakey, writing in *Family Circle* magazine (2/22/94) suggests that when eating out, children and adults should choose foods cooked in tomato sauce, or baked, broiled, grilled (dry without added fat), poached, roasted or steamed. Avoid foods described by such terms as "au gratin," "basted," "casserole," "creamed," "crispy," "fried," "in gravy," "with Hollandaise sauce," "or "sautéed." Most sauces are high in fat, especially if they contain cheese or butter.

Resources

Attwood, Charles R., M.D. *Dr. Attwood's Low-Fat Prescription for Kids.* New York: Penguin, 1995.

Barnard, Neal, M.D., with recipes by Jennifer Raymond. *Food for Life: How the New Four Food Groups Can Save Your Life.* New York: Harmony Books, 1993.

Barnard, Neal, M.D., and Jennifer Raymond. *Eat Right, Live Longer: Using the Natural Power of Foods to Age-Proof Your Body.* New York: Harmony Books, 1995.

Barnard, Neal, M.D., with Jennifer Raymond. *Foods That Fight Pain: Revolutionary New Strategies for Maximum Pain Relief.* New York: Harmony Books, 1998.

DeBakey, Michael and Antonio Grotto, Lynne Scott, John Foreyt . *The Living Heart Brand Name Shopper's Guide.* New York: Mastermedia, 1993.

DeBakey, Michael and Antonio Grotto, Lynne Scott, John Foreyt . *The Living Heart Diet.* New York: Raven, 1984.

Gross, Joy. *Raising Your Family Naturally.* New York: Lyle Stuart, Inc., 1983.

Havala, Suzanne, M.S., R.D., and Mary Clifford, R.D. *Simple, Lowfat, and Vegetarian: Unbelievably Easy Ways to Reduce the Fat in Your Meals.* Baltimore, Md.: Vegetarian Journal, 1994.

Heart-Healthy Lessons for Children. Phoenix, Ariz.: Arizona Heart Institute and Foundation, 1991.

Klaper, Michael, M.D. *Pregnancy, Children, and the Vegan Diet.* Paia, Hawaii: Gentle World, 1987. (Available from the American Vegan Society, 501 Old Harding Highway, Malaga, N.J. 08328)

Kwiterovick, Peter O., Jr., M.D. *The Johns Hopkins Complete Guide for Preventing and Reversing Heart Disease.* Rocklin, Calif.: Prima Publishing, 1993.

La Leche League International. *The Womanly Art of Breastfeeding.* New York: NAL/ Dutton, 1991.

Mangels, Reed, Ph.D., R.D. "Vegan Diet During Pregnancy, Lactation, and Childhood" (article reprint, 16 pgs.) Baltimore, Md.: *Vegetarian Journal,* 1991.

McDougall, John, M.D. and Mary A. McDougall. *The McDougall Plan.* Hampton, N.J.: New Win, 1985.

Moran, Victoria. *Get the Fat Out: 501 Simple Ways to Cut the Fat in Any Diet.* New York: Crown Trade Paperbacks, 1994.

National Research Council, *Recommended Dietary Allowances,* 10th edition. Washington, D.C.: National Academy Press, 1989.

Ornish, Dean, M.D. *Dr. Dean Ornish's Program for Reversing Heart Disease.* New York: Crown Trade Paperbacks, 1994.

————. *Eat More, Weigh Less.* New York: Harper Collins, 1993.

Robbins, John. *May All Be Fed.* New York: William Morrow and Company, 1992.

Simone, Charles B. *Cancer and Nutrition: A Ten-Point Plan to Reduce Your Risk of Getting Cancer.* Garden City Park, N.Y.: Avery Publishing Group, 1992.

Warshaw, Hope E. *Eat Out, Eat Right.* Chicago: Surrey Books, 1992.

The Wellness Encyclopedia of Good and Nutrition. University of California at Berkeley. New York: Rebus, 1992.

Internet Sites

Charles Attwood, M.D.
http://www.vegsource.org/attwood/

EarthSaveInternational
http://www.earthsave.org

Ruth Heidrich, Ph.D.
http://www.vegsource.org/heidrich/

The Jewish Vegan Lifestyle
http://www.goodnet.com/-Ljvmab/

Michael Klaper, M.D.
http://www.vegsource.org/klaper/

New Veg
http://www.newveg.av.org/

North American Vegetarian Society (NAVS)
http://www.cyberveg.org/navs

Physicians' Committee for Responsible Medicine
(PCRM)
http://www.pcrm.org/

John McDougall, M.D.
http://www.drmcdougall.com/

New Century Nutrition
http://www.paracelsian.com/NCNonline.html

International Vegetarian Union
http://www.ivu.org/

Vegetarian Central
http://www.vegetariancentral.org/

Vegetarian Resource Group
http://www.vrg.org/

Vegetarian Society U.K.
http://www.veg.org/

Vegetarian Union of North America (VUNA)
http://www.IVU.org/vuni/

Vegetarian Youth Network
http://www.geocities.com/RodeoDrive/1154

VegSource
http://www.vegsource.com/

Magazines and Newsletters

McDougall Newsletter
John McDougall, M.D.
P.O. Box 14-039
Santa Rosa, CA 954-02

Vegetarian Journal
Vegetarian Resource Group
P.O. Box 1463, Baltimore, MD 21203
(410) 366-8343

Vegetarian Times
P.O. Box 570
Oak Park, IL 60303
(708) 848-8100

Vegetarian Voice
(published by North American Vegetarian Society)
(518) 568-7970

About the Author

Charles R. Attwood, M.D., F.A.A.P., a board-certified pediatrician and Fellow of the American Academy of Pediatrics, has practiced for thirty-five years. He is the author of *Dr. Attwood's Low-Fat Prescription For Kids* (Penguin, 1995), with a Foreword by Dr. Benjamin Spock. He has written hundreds of newspaper articles on the health effects of nutrition and fitness, and co-authored a regular column with the late Dr. Benjamin Spock in the nationally respected publication, *New Century Nutrition.* Dr. Attwood also writes a regular health column in *HealthSmart* for thirty-five Louisiana newspapers, and has been a longtime writer and consultant for *Medical Economics* magazine, the nation's largest medical publication. In 1996 and '97 he worked as a consultant with Dr. Spock to revise the nutrition sections of the classic, *Dr. Spock's Baby and Child Care.*

Dr. Attwood has taken an activist role in national health and nutrition policy. For example, he, along with his colleagues, sent a document requesting the USDA to take a stronger position in favor of plant-based diets. As a result, the 1996 *U.S. Dietary Guidelines For Americans* stated for the first time that a vegetarian diet can be healthful. A similar initiative is now underway for revising the Food Pyramid. He took a strong stand against Proctor & Gamble's olestra, urging the FDA against approval of the product.

Attwood is a consultant for the Center for Science in the Public Interest in Washington, DC. He and CSPI director Michael Jacobson conducted a national press conference (February 1996) revealing that Gerber baby food was diluted with water, sugar and starches. As a result 1,500 pediatricians wrote the FDA. During the following weeks, according to *Advertising Age* magazine, Gerber's market share dropped from 80 % to 65 %. They stopped the dilution and changed their labels to "100 % fruit & 100 % vegetables." Within days, Heinz Baby Food quietly stopped their own dilution practices.

During 1995-1997, Dr. Attwood was interviewed by over 300 radio and TV stations in the U.S. and Canada, and by national networks, including CNN, ABC, CBS, FOX, Westwood One, America's Talking, PBS and NPR. He was a consultant on the Oprah Show and appeared three times on David Essel Alive.

Newspaper interviews have included *USA Today, The Washington Post, The New York Times*, as well as dozens of regional and local papers. His book was noted in *Ladies' Home Journal, Woman's World, Vegetarian Times, Publisher's Weekly, Parenting, Mothering,* and *First For Women,* among many others.

Dr. Attwood has been selected as a faculty member of the American Academy of Nutrition and a guest lecturer at Cornell University. In June of 1996 he was appointed to the Board of Advisers of EarthSave International. He was selected as one of twenty world experts to the faculty of the Second National Conference on Prevention of Coronary Heart Disease, sponsored and developed by the Cleveland Clinic at the Disney Institute in Orlando, Florida, September 4-5, 1997. He will be a keynote faculty speaker at the 12th Annual Asian Cardiology Congress in Manila, Philippines in December 1998.

His essays and articles on nutrition and heart disease have been published in the United States, Canada and Europe in English, German, and Italian. In 1998, his article, "Low-Fat Diets for Children: Safety and Practicality," will appear worldwide in the *American Journal of Cardiology.*

Dr. Charles Attwood, is the winner of the 1997 Telly Award for non-broadcast videos, as guest host of the award-winning video "Mooove Over Milk." Dr. Attwood lives and works with his wife Judy, in Crowley, Louisiana; Greenville, SC; and New York City.

Visit Dr. Attwood's web site: http://www.veg-source.org/attwood

Index

ADDITIONAL HEALTH TITLES FROM HOHM PRESS

YOUR BODY CAN TALK: How to Listen to What Your Body Knows and Needs Through Simple Muscle Testing
by Susan L. Levy, D.C. and Carol Lehr, M.A.

Imagine having a diagnostic tool so sensitive that it could immediately tell you: • exactly how much protein...or fat...Your Body needs...• precisely which vitamins and minerals are needed in Your Diet...• what particular factors in the environment are depleting Your Vital Energy...• what hidden allergies you may have • which organs in your body are weakened due to over-stress • or anything else related to your health and well-being. You Already Have This Tool...at your own fingertips. Dr. Levy and Carol Lehr present clear instructions in *simple muscle testing*, together with over 25 simple tests for how to use it for specific problems or disease conditions. Special chapters deal with health problems specific to women (especially PMS and Menopause) and problems specific to men (like stress, heart disease, and prostate difficulties). Contains over 30 diagrams, plus a complete Index and Resource Guide.

Paper, 350 pages, $19.95, ISBN: 0-934252-68-8

• • •

NATURAL HEALING WITH HERBS
by Humbart "Smokey" Santillo, N.D.
Foreword by Robert S. Mendelsohn, M.D.

Dr. Santillo's first book, and Hohm Press' long-standing bestseller, is a classic handbook on herbal and naturopathic treatment. Acclaimed as the most comprehensive work of its kind, *Natural Healing With Herbs* details (in layperson's terms) the properties and uses of 120 of the most common herbs and lists comprehensive therapies for more than 140 common ailments. All in alphabetical order for quick reference.
Includes special sections on: • Diagnosis • How to make herbal remedies • The nature of health and disease • Diet and detoxification • Homeopathy... and more

Over 150,000 copies in print.
Paper, 408 pages, $16.95, ISBN: 0-934252-08-4

TO ORDER PLEASE SEE ACCOMPANYING ORDER FORM OR CALL 1-800-381-2700 TO PLACE YOUR ORDER NOW.

ADDITIONAL HEALTH TITLES FROM HOHM PRESS

FOOD ENZYMES: THE MISSING LINK TO RADIANT HEALTH
by Humbart "Smokey" Santillo, N.D.

Immune system health is a subject of concern for everyone today. This book explains how the body's immune system, as well as every other human metabolic function, requires enzymes in order to work properly. Food enzyme supplementation is more essential today than ever before, since stress, unhealthy food, and environmental pollutants readily deplete them from the body. Humbart Santillo's breakthrough book presents the most current research in this field, and encourages simple, straightforward steps for how to make enzyme supplementation a natural addition to a nutrition-conscious lifestyle.

Special sections on: • Longevity and disease • The value of raw food and juicing • Detoxification • Prevention of allergies and candida • Sports and nutrition

Over 200,000 copies in print.

Paper, 108 pages, U.S. $7.95, ISBN: 0-934252-40-8 (English)

Now available in Spanish language version.

Paper, 108 pages, U.S. $6.95, ISBN: 0-934252-49-1 (Spanish)

■ Audio version of Food Enzymes
2 cassette tapes, 150 minutes, U.S. $17.95, ISBN: 0-934252-29-7

• • •

INTUITIVE EATING: EveryBody's Guide to Vibrant Health and Lifelong Vitality Through Food
by Humbart "Smokey" Santillo, N.D.

The natural voice of the body has been drowned out by the shouts of addictions, over-consumption, and devitalized and preserved foods. Millions battle the scale daily, experimenting with diets and nutritional programs, only to find their victories short-lived at best, confusing and demoralizing at worst. *Intuitive Eating* offers an alternative—a tested method for: • strengthening the immune system • natural weight loss • increasing energy • making the transition from a degenerative diet to a regenerative diet • slowing the aging process.

Paper, 450 pages, $16.95, ISBN: 0-934252-27-0

TO ORDER PLEASE SEE ACCOMPANYING ORDER FORM OR CALL 1-800-381-2700 TO PLACE YOUR ORDER NOW.

ADDITIONAL HEALTH TITLES FROM HOHM PRESS

ARE YOU GETTING IT 5 TIMES A DAY?
Fruits and Vegetables
by Sydney H. Crackower, M.D., Barry A. Bohn, M.D. and
Rodney Langlinais, Reg. Pharmacist

The evidence is irrefutable. Research from around the world, and from the American
Cancer Society and the National Cancer Institute in the U.S. agree ... 5 servings of
nature's disease fighters—raw fruits and vegetables—would markedly reduce
cancer...stroke...and heart disease, the leading killers of our times. Fresh fruits and
vegetables, as well as an intelligently pursued regimen of antioxidants, live enzymes
and high fiber are the nutritional basics of good health. This concise and
straightforward book will give you all the background research and practical steps
you need to start getting it today!

Paper, 78 pages, $ 6.95, ISBN: 0-934252-35-1

• • •

■ *HERBS, NUTRITION AND HEALING ;* AUDIO CASSETTE SERIES
by Dr. Humbart "Smokey" Santillo, N.D.

Santillo's most comprehensive seminar series. Topics covered in-depth include: •
the history of herbology • specific preparation of herbs for tinctures, salves,
concentrates, etc. • herbal dosages in both acute and chronic illnesses • use of
cleansing and transition diets • treating colds and flu... and more.

4 cassettes, 330 minutes, $40.00, ISBN: 0-934252-22-X

• • •

■ *NATURE HEALS FROM WITHIN;* AUDIO CASSETTE SERIES
by Dr. Humbart "Smokey" Santillo, N.D.

How to take the next step in improving your life and health through nutrition. Topics
include: • The innate wisdom of the body. • The essential role of elimination and
detoxification • Improving digestion • How "transition dieting" will take off the
weight—for good! • The role of heredity, diet, and prevention in health • How to
overcome tiredness, improve your immune system and live longer...and happier.

1 cassette, $8.95, ISBN: 0-934252-66-1

TO ORDER PLEASE SEE ACCOMPANYING ORDER FORM
OR CALL 1-800-381-2700 TO PLACE YOUR ORDER NOW.

ADDITIONAL HEALTH TITLES FROM HOHM PRESS

■ *LIVE SEMINAR ON FOOD ENZYMES*; AUDIO CASSETTE SERIES
by Dr. Humbart "Smokey" Santillo, N.D.

An in-depth discussion of the properties of food enzymes, describing their valuable use to maintain vitality, immunity, health and longevity. A must for anyone interested in optimal health. Complements all the information in the book.

1 cassette, $8.95, ISBN: 0-934252-29-7

• • •

■ *FRUITS AND VEGETABLES—The Basis of Health*; AUDIO CASSETTE SERIES
by Dr. Humbart "Smokey" Santillo, N.D.

Juicing of fruits and vegetables is one of the fastest and most efficient ways to supply the body with the raw food nutrients and enzymes needed to maintain optimal health. Explains the essential difference between a live food diet, which heals the body, and degenerative foods, which weaken the immune system and cause disease. Recipes included.

1 cassette, $8.95, ISBN: 0-934252-65-3

• • •

■ *WEIGHT-LOSS SEMINAR*; AUDIO CASSETTE SERIES
by Dr. Humbart "Smokey" Santillo, N.D.

"The healthiest people in the world know the secret of weight loss," says Santillo in this candid, practical, and information-based seminar. "If your body is getting what it needs, the appetite automatically turns off!" The reason for overweight is that we are starving ourselves to death, based on the improper balance of nutrients from our current food sources. This seminar explains the worthlessness of most dietary regimens and explodes many common myths about weight gain. Santillo stresses: • The essential distinction between "good" fats and "bad" fats • The necessity for protein and how to use it efficiently • How to get our primary vitamins and minerals from food • How to ease into becoming an "intuitive eater" so that the body is always getting what it knows it needs.

1 cassette, $8.95, ISBN: 0-934252-75-0

TO ORDER PLEASE SEE ACCOMPANYING ORDER FORM OR CALL 1-800-381-2700 TO PLACE YOUR ORDER NOW.

ADDITIONAL HEALTH TITLES FROM HOHM PRESS

10 ESSENTIAL FOODS
by Lalitha Thomas

Lalitha has done for food what she did with such wit and wisdom for herbs in her best-selling *10 Essential Herbs*. This new book presents 10 ordinary, but *essential* and great-tasting foods that can: • Strengthen a weakened immune system • Rebalance brain chemistry • Fight cancer and other degenerative diseases • Help you lose weight, simply and naturally.

Carrots, broccoli, almonds, grapefruit and six other miracle foods will enhance your health when used regularly and wisely. Lalitha gives in-depth nutritional information plus flamboyant and good-humored stories about these foods, based on her years of health and nutrition counseling. Each chapter contains easy and delicious recipes, tips for feeding kids and helpful hints for managing your food dollar. A bonus section supports the use of 10 Essential Snacks.

"This book's focus is squarely on target: fruits, vegetables and whole grains— everything comes in the right natural proportions."—Charles Attwood, M.D., F.A.A.P.; author, *Dr. Attwoods Low-Fat Prescription for Kids* (Viking).

Paper, 300 pages, $16.95, ISBN: 0-934252-74-2

• • •

THE MELATONIN AND AGING SOURCEBOOK
by Dr. Roman Rozencwaig, M.D. and Dr. Hasnain Walji, Ph.D.

"This is the most comprehensive reference on melatonin, yet published. It is an indispensable tool for those scientists, researchers, and physicians engaged in anti-aging therapeutics." —Dr. Ronald Klatz, President, American Academy of Anti-aging Medicing

This book covers the latest research on the pineal...control of aging, melatonin and sleep, melatonin and immunity, melatonin's role in cancer treatment, antioxidant qualities of melatonin, dosages, counter indications, quality control, and use with other drugs, melatonin application to heart disease, Alzheimer's, diabetes, stress, major depression, seasonal affective disorders, AIDS, SIDS, cataracts, autism...and many other conditions.

Cloth, 220 pages, $79.95, ISBN: 0-934252-73-4

TO ORDER PLEASE SEE ACCOMPANYING ORDER FORM OR CALL 1-800-381-2700 TO PLACE YOUR ORDER NOW.

RETAIL ORDER FORM FOR HOHM PRESS HEALTH BOOKS

Name_____ Phone ( )_____

Street Address or P.O. Box _____

City _____ State _____ Zip Code _____

	QTY	TITLE	ITEM PRICE	TOTAL PRICE	
1		**10 ESSENTIAL FOODS**	$16.95		
2		**10 ESSENTIAL HERBS**	$16.95		
3		**ARE YOU GETTING IT 5 TIMES A DAY?**	$6.95		
4		**DHEA: The Ultimate Rejuvenating Hormone**	$9.95		
5		**FOOD ENZYMES/ENGLISH**	$7.95		
6		**FOOD ENZYMES/SPANISH**	$6.95		
7		**FOOD ENZYMES BOOK/AUDIO**	$17.95		
8		**FRUITS & VEGETABLES/AUDIO**	$8.95		
9		**HERBS, NUTRITION AND HEALING/AUDIO**	$40.00		
10		**INTUITIVE EATING**	$16.95		
11		**LIVE SEMINAR ON FOOD ENZYMES/AUDIO**	$8.95		
12		**THE MELATONIN AND AGING SOURCEBOOK**	$79.95		
13		**NATURAL HEALING WITH HERBS**	$16.95		
14		**NATURE HEALS FROM WITHIN/AUDIO**	$8.95		
15		**THE VEGETARIAN DOCTOR SPEAKS OUT**	$14.95		
16		**WEIGHT LOSS SEMINAR/AUDIO**	$8.95		
17		**YOUR BODY CAN TALK: How to Listen...**	$19.95		

SURFACE SHIPPING CHARGES

1st book $4.00
Each additional item $1.00

SUBTOTAL:

SHIPPING: (see below)

TOTAL:

SHIP MY ORDER

☐ Surface U.S. Mail—Priority
☐ 2nd-Day Air (Mail + $5.00)
☐ UPS (Mail + $2.00)
☐ Next-Day Air (Mail + $15.00)

METHOD OF PAYMENT:

☐ Check or M.O.   Payable to Hohm Press, P.O. Box 2501, Prescott, AZ 86302
☐ Call 1-800-381-2700 to place your credit card order
☐ Or call 1-520-717-1779 to fax your credit card order
☐ Information for Visa/MasterCard order only:

Card #_____–_____–_____–_____   Expiration Date _____

ORDER NOW! Call 1-800-381-2700 or fax your order to 1-520-717-1779.
(Remember to include your credit card information.)